Vital Healing

of related interest

Celestial Healing
Energy, Mind & Spirit in Traditional Medicine of China and East &
Southeast Asia With Treatments for Common Conditions – Greater
China
Marc S. Micozzi with Kevin Ergil, MA, MS, LAc and Laurel Gabler, PhD
ISBN 978 1 84819 060 3

Wan's Clinical Application of Chinese Medicine
Scientific Practice of Diagnosis, Treatment and Therapeutic Monitoring
Giorgio Repeti, LAc, with Marc S. Micozzi, MD, PhD
ISBN 978 1 84819 047 4

Contemporary Ayurvedic Medicine
Hari Sharma, Christopher S. Clark and Marc S. Micozzi
ISBN 978 1 84819 069 6

Chinese Medical Qigong
Editor in Chief: Tianjun Liu, OMD
Foreword by Marc Micozzi, MD, PhD
Associate Editor in Chief: Kevin W. Chen, PhD
ISBN 978 1 84819 023 8

Vital Healing

Energy, Mind and Spirit in Traditional Medicines
of India, Tibet and the Middle East – Middle Asia

Marc S. Micozzi, MD, PhD

with Donald McCown, MAMS, MSS
and
Mones Abu-Asab, PhD (Unani),
Hakima Amri, PhD (Unani),
Kevin Ergil, MA, MS, LAc (Tibet),
Howard Hall, PsyD, PhD (Sufi),
Hari Sharma, MD (Maharishi Ayurveda),
Kenneth G. Zysk, Dphil, PhD (Ayurveda and Siddha)

SINGING
DRAGON

LONDON AND PHILADELPHIA

First published in 2011
by Singing Dragon
an imprint of Jessica Kingsley Publishers
116 Pentonville Road
London N1 9JB, UK
and
400 Market Street, Suite 400
Philadelphia, PA 19106, USA

www.singing-dragon.com

Copyright © Marc S. Micozzi 2011

Library of Congress Cataloging in Publication Data
A CIP catalog record for this book is available from the Library of Congress

British Library Cataloguing in Publication Data
A CIP catalogue record for this book is available from the British Library

ISBN 978 1 84819 045 0

Printed and bound in the United States by
Thomson-Shore, Inc.

Contents

Chronological Phases of Indian and Middle Asian Medicine, with Sanskrit, Vedic, Buddhist, Muslim, Unani, British Colonial, Nationalist and New Age Influences

Indus River Valley Civilization	2500 BCE	Developed public health and medical practices; exchange with Mesopotamia
Vedic Period	1500–100 BCE	Vedic texts; first medical classics
	1100–700 BCE	Brahmana and Upanishads; Sushruta, founder of Indian anatomy and surgery
Buddha	560–480 BCE	Jivaka, Indian surgeon under Buddha
Nanda Dynasty	350–320 BCE	Development of Ayurvedic medicine; Greek observations and documentation of human and veterinary medicine in India
Alexander the Great	327–325 BCE	
Maurya Dynasty	320–185 BCE	
Sunga Dynasty	185–75 BCE	
Kusana Dynasty	1–300 CE	Samhita of Caraka
Gupta Dynasty	320–500 CE	Peak of Ayurvedic medicine
Reign of Harsha	606–647 CE	Vagbhata's *Astangdahrdayasamhita*
Conquest of Sind by Muslims	712 CE	
Local Princely States	800–1200 CE	Madhava's *Treatise on Etiology* Vranda's and Vanagsena's *Therapeutics*

Muslim Conquest of India	1200–1300 CE	Introduction of Unani (Greco-Arabic) medicine
Sultanate of Delhi	1300–1500 CE	
Khalji Dynasty	1290–1320 CE	Sarngadhara's *Treatise on Medicine*; Ayurvedic concept of circulation
Tughluq Dynasty	1320–1413 CE	Diya Mohammed's *Majmu'e Diya'e* Madanapala's *Materia Medica of Ayurveda*
Sayyid and Lodi Dynasties	1414–1526 CE	
Mogul Dynasty	1500–1700 CE	Golden Age of Unani medicine; Bhavamishra's *Treatise on Ayurveda*
British Empire	1700–1947 CE	Introduction of Western medicine; recovery of traditional medicines
Indian Republic	1947–	Research on traditional medicine; clinical and pharmacological studies
Maharishi Ayurveda	1967–	Rejuvenation of traditional Ayurveda; introduction of twentieth-century physics and "consciousness model" of Ayurveda

Preface

As a physician and anthropologist I have seen many books on the medical traditions of Asia which are known to anthropologists as ethnomedicine and to physicians as complementary or alternative medicine. Academic dissertations are written to show the differences between different traditions. But what has struck me are the similarities among them.

Many books have been written about Chinese medicine, fewer on Ayurvedic medicine of India, and very few on Tibetan or Unani medicine, or Sufi healing. I am aware of no book that has concentrated on, and encompassed, all of these lesser known Middle Asian ethnomedical traditions together. To be able to write about all of them in continuity has been a challenge and a joy. And I have tried to show the influence of Chinese medicine on these traditions, and vice versa, without writing another book about Chinese medicine.

Another striking aspect of these lesser known traditions is how, in their ancient wisdom—as much as knowledge—about body, mind and spirit, they seem to anticipate modern thinking about the deepest, most fundamental nature of the cosmos and of reality itself. While these insights were made possible in the West in the twentieth century only by quantum mechanics and Einstein's theory of relativity, this ancient Eastern knowledge of health and healing seems to intuit it all through its understanding of energy and spirit as embodied in the human being.

I would like to acknowledge the many colleagues who have helped open the doors about this ancient knowledge in a most profound way through years of disciplined scholarship, research and practice in fields once somewhat obscure but now made popular by the burgeoning consumer movement of complementary/alternative medicine, from A to Z: Mones Abu-Asab, PhD, Amy Ai, PhD, Hakima Amri, PhD, Claire Cassidy, PhD, LAc, Christopher Clark, MD, Kevin Ergil, MA, MS, LAc, Marnae Ergil, MA, MS, LAc, Howard Hall, PhD, PsyD, John Ives, PhD, Michael Jawer, Wayne Jonas, MD, Donald McCown, MAMS, MSS, LSW, David Mayor, MA, BAc, MBAcCL, Rhadheshyam Miryala, MD, Hari Sharma, MD, FRCPC, Devna Singh, MD, Georgia Tetlow, MSW, MD, Christine Vlahos, MSPT, and Kenneth Zysk, PhD, DPhil.

I also thank Jessica Kingsley for her personal, timely and thoughtful consideration of this work in progress. She helped bring order out of chaos for this book, much like some of the characters mentioned therein, such as Einstein, Eddington and Heisenberg, did for the universe (or perhaps vice versa).

Chapter 1

Vital Healing

Body, Mind, and Spirit

Mind, healing, and consciousness

The healing traditions we encounter in this book consider spiritual consciousness to be of primary importance in maintaining optimal health, emphasizing meditation and movement practices and other modalities that foster integrated (holistic) functioning of the nervous system.

All these healing traditions have developed sophisticated theoretical frameworks that provide insight into the functioning of body, mind and spirit together.

- Understanding of *mind–body type* is essential to diagnosis and treatment.

- Emphasis is placed on the therapeutic effects of diet and healthy digestion, as well as techniques to balance behavior and emotions.

- Extensive *materia medica* describe the therapeutic use of medicinal plants.

- There is detailed understanding of biological rhythms, which form the basis for daily and seasonal behavioral routines.

- All of these approaches can be seen to strengthen the immune system and homeostatic mechanisms with our modern understanding of human medicine.

Getting the whole picture

Ancient medical texts of this Middle Asian realm typically begin with a thorough description of strategies of prevention before discussing modalities for treatment. While we make important distinctions in Western medicine between public health strategies for preventing disease, and medical interventions for treating acute disease, and for chronic disease—generally speaking, the holistic approaches of Asian medical systems find that the same techniques that help prevent disease are also used to treat diseases when they occur, since they deal with the causes and not just the symptoms.

In addition to preventive techniques, these traditions offer holistic theories for disease prevention and health promotion. For diagnosis and treatment, there are large numbers of procedures and protocols, including sets of non-invasive diagnostic techniques which overcome some serious limitations of Western (allopathic) medicine. For example, in the United States today, functional diseases, such as irritable bowel syndrome and poor digestion, chronic headache, chronic fatigue, menstrual dysfunction, account for approximately one-half of patient visits to family practitioners. Western medicine, however, lacks well-developed theories or methods of treatment for these disorders.

When the cure is worse than the disease

Sir Francis Bacon, the sixteenth-century British philosopher and scientist, recognized circumstances when "the cure is worse than the disease." In addition to missing the whole picture of the patient, another major area of concern with modern Western medicine is iatrogenic diseases (physician caused diseases, from the Greek *iatros*, for physician). At the outset of the twenty-first century, with all its medical miracles and biotech promises, these physician-caused diseases are estimated to be the third leading cause of death in the United States (Starfield 2000). A study of hospitalized patients found that over one-third are afflicted with iatrogenic illnesses. At least one serious "adverse event" (another term for iatrogenic occurrences) resulting from inappropriate care lengthened the hospital stay of nearly one-fifth of hospital patients (Andrews *et al.* 1997) and nearly one-eighth of adverse events led to death (Berwick and Leape 1999).

The co-author of the last-listed study, Donald Berwick, was appointed to the position of Director of the Center for Medicare and Medicaid Services in the United States in 2010, and it is hoped that his awareness of these problems will help improve the safety as well as decrease the costs of medical therapies. Dr. Berwick has confronted the reality of health care rationing, but advocates sensible rationing, rather than the blind, de facto rationing that occurs today dictated solely by health insurance company profits and problems with access. Based upon studies like these, it can be estimated that one-third of health care is unnecessary and even counterproductive. If the alternative medical treatments that have already been proven safe, effective and cost-effective were used appropriately, one could increase this estimate to two-thirds of present-day mainstream health care (Micozzi 1998). The adverse events of mainstream practices are presently accepted as known complications of treatment, and managing these expected events is factored into the high cost of medical care.

A large percentage of iatrogenic illnesses are the result of side effects from drugs. Adverse drug reactions have become the fourth leading cause of death in the United States (Lazarou, Pomeranz and Corey 1998).

Losing the war on cancer

To consider one example, Western biomedical approaches to cancer treatment have severe side effects, and some anti-tumor drugs and radiation treatments actually contribute to the development of new cancers. Physicians of Sir Francis

Bacon's era might recognize the medieval treatments of "burning, cutting and poisoning" reflected in the modern cancer treatments of, respectively, radiation (burning), surgery (cutting) and chemotherapy (poisoning), where the hope is that the treatments are more harmful to the cancer than they are to the patient. Many Asian medical modalities have been proven effective in reducing the side effects of several of these treatments, such as acupuncture for chemotherapy-induced nausea and pain, as well as ginger for this nausea. Research has also shown that some herbal preparations, including many from the vast Ayurvedic pharmacopeia (see Chapter 3), may reduce cancer growth directly and even induce cancer cells to return to normal cells (said to help them "remember" the right path).

Magic bullets and friendly fire

In terms of infectious disease and epidemics, the Western approach of using antibiotics also has inherent limitations and risks caused by the process of natural selection that produces new, resistant strains of microbes. As a result, overreliance on antibiotics has fostered the development of serious new infectious diseases such as MRSA (Methicillin Resistant Staphylococcus Aureus, and so-called "flesh-eating bacteria"), chloroquine-resistant malaria, and other modern plagues. A similar process may also occur with cancer, as powerful chemopreventive agents select for the survival of those cancer cells which can no longer be treated by chemotherapy at all, no matter how toxic they are to the patient.

During the nineteenth century, Western medicine sought drugs that could kill infectious bacteria without harming the host. This goal was critical, as the drugs once used to treat infections, such as lead, mercury and arsenic compounds, while killing the bacteria, were extremely harmful if not lethal for the patients. Oliver Wendell Holmes, at an address to the Massachusetts Medical Society (publisher of the influential *New England Journal of Medicine*) said in 1860, "if the entire materia medica as currently practiced could be sunk to the bottom of the sea, it would be all the better for mankind, and all the worse for the fishes."

Paul Ehrlich's discovery of Salvarsan in 1906 provided a "magic bullet" that killed the bacteria (in that case, syphilis) without seriously harming the patient. (Although we now know that antibiotics also kill many beneficial bacteria in the intestinal tract—so-called "pro-biotics"—and disrupt the internal environment for digestion). This discovery was soon followed by the development of true antibiotics which, instead of killing bacteria like antiseptics, simply stop bacterial reproduction until the patient's own immune system naturally overcomes the infection. This approach allows the immune system to work naturally, as it does when infection produces a fever, by slowing bacterial growth until the body naturally overcomes the infection (Figure 1.1).

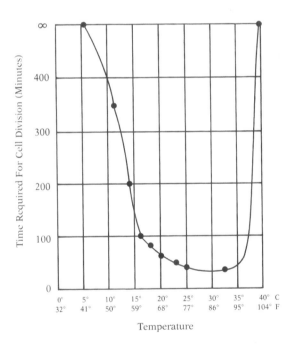

Figure 1.1 Relation between rate of cell division for bacteria (Bacillus Sp.) and temperature. Above normal body temperatures the time required for bacteria to divide and multiply rapidly approaches infinity, thus demonstrating the natural bacteriostatic effect of fever

Source: Data from Encyclopedia Brittanica, 1954 edition

Early antibiotics were also natural in another sense—like penicillin, they are made by other microbes in the environment as they compete with fellow microbes to grow, again through the process of natural selection. By the same process of natural selection, the success and (over)use of antibiotics during the twentieth century led to the development of antibiotic resistance, generating many new and dangerous bacterial strains, resistant to antibiotic treatment—turning "magic bullets" into "friendly fire." In the presence of antibiotics, bacteria adapt by creating offspring that are immune to the effects of the antiobiotic. Fortunately, bacteria are unable to develop resistance to the complex *mixtures* of active constituents that occur naturally in herbal preparations. For example, the crude extract of the cinchona bark, original source of quinine, remains potent against chloroquine-resistant malaria.

We will see that virtually all traditional medical systems, including those of Middle Asia in this book, have learned to grow plants that provide complex mixtures of biologically active ingredients to treat infections found within their own natural environments.

The traditional medical modalties which strengthen immunity in harmony with homeostatic mechanisms are like "natural antibiotics." Looking back at the triumphs and pitfalls of twentieth-century medicine, we can begin to understand where the more holistic approaches of the ancient traditions as exemplified by Middle Asia offer advantages by being more aligned with the nature of the body and with Nature itself. But there is yet another dimension that has been revealed to us by twentieth-century fundamental physics and quantum mechanics. For those who are not mathematically inclined, or who are intimidated by "hard science," please do not skip ahead to the next chapter, because the complex mathematics and equations of these early twentieth-century geniuses have ultimately led back to a very human philosophy about the nature of reality which can be appreciated by everyone. And it is the philosophy, not the mathematics, that is now described in the next section.

From medieval physick to modern physics

During the times of Sir Francis Bacon and Sir Isaac Newton, medicine was known in English as physic, often spelled physick. What we call physics today was studied by Isaac Newton as mechanics and optics, which had continued to be investigated by Muslim physicians in the Middle East and Middle Asia. They kept the lights on during the long, dark, medieval period in Europe of the Middle Ages—until European investigations resumed during the Age of Enlightenment, reaching England and Scotland with full illumination in the late seventeenth and eighteenth centuries.

Newton would ponder the effects of gravity when an apple fell and hit him on the head while sitting under an apple tree, ultimately leading to his formulation of classical, Newtonian mechanics. Mechanics could explain why the apple fell, but not why the apple existed or why Newton was thinking about it in the first place—questions left to another age. One answer as to why Newton was sitting under the apple tree is that he had escaped to the country to avoid the effects of a plague epidemic, causing him never to complete his doctoral studies at Oxford University (perhaps ultimately a great benefit to posterity).

Until the early twentieth century, the field of physics remained based on Newton's solid (like the apple), mechanical, materialist approach to the natural world. The allopathic or Western medical paradigm, developed in the nineteenth century, is based on this mechanical physics of materialism; it views the body as a complex machine. However, discoveries by twentieth-century physicists expanded our worldview beyond materialism and, further, uncovered a fundamental role for consciousness in the physical world. Because the nature and importance of consciousness are not usually considered in allopathic medicine, we must turn to these insights of twentieth-century physics to provide a useful background for understanding vital healing— and what appears to have already been known by the ancient physicians of Middle Asia.

According to the materialist theory that delimited physics until the early 1900s, the universe is made up of solid, discrete bits of matter. These particles affect each other only through direct interactions. Four basic principles support this common-sense, Newtonian view of everyday physical reality:

1. *Solid matter*: the world is fundamentally made up of solid material objects, the building blocks of nature.

2. *Strict causality*: change in motion of one object can be caused only by direct interaction with another object.

3. *Locality*: interactions between particles can occur only through collisions or through influences radiated through the electromagnetic or gravitational fields at the speed of light, or less; no non-local interaction can occur.

4. *Reductionism*: large systems in nature—including, in principle, the human body and even the entire universe—can be understood completely by understanding the properties and local, causal interactions of their smallest discrete components.

Further, this materialist theory considers the consciousness of the scientist to be entirely separate from the material objects being studied. The knower (consciousness) and the known (object) are thought to exist in completely distinct domains. This separation is thought to be the basis of "objective" science. This "fact" was challenged by Werner Heisenberg a century ago when he proved that the act of observation by the observer fundamentally influences the phenomenon being observed at the microscopic level. The Heisenberg "Uncertainty Principle" has become a foundation of quantum mechanics and the new physics. Throughout the history of science the separation of consciousness from the apparently material world had led to theoretical difficulties. For example, if consciousness is completely separate from matter, it is difficult to explain how consciousness could arise from the purely mechanical interactions of solid matter within the brain.

Quantum forces

During the twentieth century the terms of this discussion were changed forever by the fundamental discoveries of quantum physics. Experiments performed in the first quarter of the twentieth century indicated that subatomic particles, the supposed building blocks of nature, did not appear to be composed of solid matter. In some of these experiments, particles behaved as if they were waves. While the Nobel Prize had been awarded to nineteenth-century British physicist J. J. Thompson for his discovery that electrons are particles, a generation later, it was awarded to his son George P. Thompson for *his* discovery that electrons are waves.

It was observed that electrons take instantaneous, discontinuous quantum jumps from one atomic orbit to another, with no intervening time and no travel through space—an impossible act for a classic particle. It also was shown that an individual subatomic particle cannot have both a precise position and a precise momentum simultaneously (the "uncertainty" of Heisenberg's Uncertainty Principle), a situation that could not apply to a solid material particle. Finally, it was found that electrons can, with predictable regularity, tunnel through a solid barrier that, classically, would be impenetrable.

On the basis of these findings, the basic principles of quantum mechanics (often known as the Copenhagen Interpretation) correct the materialist worldview:

1. *No solid matter*: this interpretation accepts the scientific findings (wave/particle, quantum jumps, uncertainty, tunneling) that contradict the notion of solid matter.

2. *No strict causality*: precise predictions for individual subatomic particles are impossible; thus, quantum mechanics loses the ability to trace causal relations among individual particles.

3. *No locality*: quantum mechanical equations indicate that two particles, once they have interacted, are instantaneously connected, even across astronomical distances—defying the insistence upon local connections in classic materialism.

4. *No reductionism*: if apparently separate particles actually are connected non-locally, a reductionist view based on isolated particles is untenable.

Wonderful, wonderful Copenhagen

This new view of reality, united under what became known as the Copenhagen Interpretation, was not able to be put to experimental test for decades, leaving some physicists unconvinced that solidity, causality, locality, and reductionism had to be abandoned. During and despite World War I, a remarkable correspondence was kept up by Sir Arthur Eddington in England and Albert Einstein, who was working with Heisenberg, Fritz Haber, Max Born, Max Planck and others in Germany. This correspondence led Eddington with his colleague Frank Watson Dyson to form the Royal Astronomical Society, to perform observations during a total eclipse of the sun in 1919 on the island of Principe, off the coast of Africa, showing that the gravity of the sun bends light emitted by distant stars and thus providing the first demonstration of Einstein's Theory of Relativity. By the 1980s a number of different experiments produced results that consistently contradicted the theories of materialism (often called local realism) and consistently confirmed the predictions of quantum mechanics and relativity. These famous experiments, tested Bell's theorem, and found that, much to Einstein's chagrin, once two particles have interacted, they are instantaneously correlated non-locally, over arbitrarily vast distances—an impossibility in materialism.

The quantum enigma

Since its inception quantum mechanics has had a problem with consciousness. This problem persists, in spite of being the most rigorously tested theory in all of science. Furthermore no test ever performed has ever failed to agree completely with the theory. So, where is the problem?

Although quantum mechanics has long been applied to much of our daily lives from computers to MRIs (magnetic resonance imaging), there is an aspect that is counterintuitive and paradoxical. This enigma is best illustrated with light in what is called the double-slit experiment. Light has a dual (and paradoxical) nature. It can be either a wave or a "particle" (photon) and Nobel Prizes have been awarded for demonstrating not only that light is a wave, but also that light is a particle.

Einstein's own Nobel Prize was awarded for his description of the photo-electric effect whereby a photon of light is like an electrical impulse but at the same time it can behave like a particle. Which of these states in which light exists at any moment is dependent on our conscious observation. How can this be? The evidence has never been refuted and, in fact, the more sophisticated we become in our experiments and tests, the more entrenched and mysterious this phenomenon becomes.

A double-slit interference experiment can be done in the following way (as this is not a book or chapter on quantum mechanics, as promised, we will skip some of the details). Light is shone into the back of two open boxes with slits on the front sides. On the wall opposite the slits, on the other side from the light source, is a projector screen. No light can reach this screen except that which comes through the slits. If the slits are narrow enough and spaced properly, the waves of light come out the slits and, because they are made of waves with high (peaks) and low (valleys) points, the waves can interact and interfere with each other in a fashion analogous to waves on water. The light spreads out from the two slits and the waves interact where they strike the screen. Where two peaks reach the screen at the same point there is a light band. Where two valleys reach the screen at the same point, there is a shadow, as no light has reached this point. What one sees, as demonstrated all the time in high school physics courses around the world, is a series of light and dark stripes, or "interference patterns." This behavior is considered definitive evidence for the wave nature of light.

However, the experiment can also be run so that only a single "packet" of light exists in *both* boxes (this is the part we are skipping over but this experiment has been done... many times). When this procedure is followed, the wave-like interference pattern is still generated, demonstrating that light is a wave and that the wave of energy was distributed in both boxes. However, if there are photon detectors in both boxes, and we *observe* them while the experiment is running, only *one* of the detectors will react and a photon (a quantum of light energy) will be found in only one box. Furthermore, the interference pattern will not appear because there is no longer a wave of light. The wave function is said to "collapse" and form the photon. If you find this confusing, you are in good company. No one has been able to adequately explain this undisputed phenomenon called *complementarity*. It is important to note that no physicist disputes this phenomenon but there is considerable controversy as to how to interpret it. Many simply choose to ignore it and its implications. (To the extent that the *mechanisms* of much of complementary medicine become understood to be based on this *quantum enigma* it may some day be labeled *complementarity medicine*.)

If you repeat this experiment many times, it always comes out one of two ways. If there is no photon detector, then we see the wave nature of light. If there are photon counters in both boxes that we *observe*, then we see only photons and no wave. Furthermore, the probability of finding the photon in one box or the other is exactly 50:50. It was this phenomenon that drove Einstein to try to wish it away by saying that "God does not play dice." The reader will have noted that we used *italics* when describing the act of *observation*. This is where consciousness comes in. As strange as this sounds, the collapsing of the wave function is dependent not only on the presence of the instruments but also on our conscious awareness of their output. This phenomenon is demonstrated elegantly in the work of Walborn and colleagues on a phenomenon called *quantum erasure*.

These studies address another aspect of quantum physics called *entanglement*. It appears that the universe makes most, if not all, things in pairs. Thus, it is possible to entangle two photons such that they have paired aspects of their quantum natures (again we are glossing over the technical details, but entanglement at the photon level has been demonstrated repeatedly). Two photons thus entangled have a very strange property: without any detectable form of energy transfer or communication and in a distance-independent manner, whatever is done to one photon *immediately*, without time delay and no matter the distance separating them, affects the other entangled photon. This is not a causal effect. Observation and the observer do not cause the effect. Rather, the effect is said to be a *non-local connectivity* or non-local correlation.

Where does that leave us? Light has a dual nature and which of its two natures it demonstrates depends upon *how we look at it.* When photons, and apparently other very small quantum particles, are entangled, they remain entangled regardless of the distance between them. Furthermore, whatever happens to one is immediately reflected in the other without any time delay and with no detectable or explainable form of energy or information transfer. This instantaneous interaction at potentially infinite distance obviously travels far faster than the speed of light, if "travel" is the right word at all—challenging Einstein's postulate that nothing can travel faster than the speed of light—unless through "worm holes," or along "superstring" fields, at the proverbial "(time) warp speed."

We may conclude, as do some physicists, that these observations demonstrate interaction among consciousness and energy and matter that appears to extend beyond even currently understood principles of physics, and that there are ways to transfer information that are independent of distance and through means that physics has not yet determined.

This incorporation of quantum physics into discussion on body-mind-spirit medicine of ancient Middle Asia provides a possible explanation for some of the empirical observations, anomalies and hallmarks of these healing traditions. In addition to helping to explain the role of consciousness in healing, and energy medicine in particular, quantum mechanics and physics may explain some of the anomalous observations that have been made in aspects of this medicine such as *distant healing.*

Most forms of energy obey an *inverse square law.* That is, the effect or force drops as an inverse square of the distance. Quantum effects do not show this drop off with distance. Further, all other energies exert their influence either at or below the speed of light. Quantum effects, like many phenomena in vital healing, seem to happen immediately without an appreciable time delay. Thus, two of the anomalous aspects of this vital healing, *independence of time and distance*, are also observed in quantum effects. In this way we may explain the exchange of healing information, or "subtle energy", between healer and patient from a distance.

We are not alone in making this connection. Cyril W. Smith has postulated that the body functions as a macroscopic quantum system (Smith 1998, 2011). This idea may be applicable to related fields of energy medicine. In his 2003 article, Smith's data suggest that the acupuncture meridian system, for example (see Chapter 2), is made of quantum domains and networks (Smith 2003). The proposition that consciousness and intention are connected through quantum mechanical means to the body-mind-spirit healing potential has been proposed by others.

However, there are problems with this hypothesis. Specifically, quantum effects have been demonstrated only on the extremely small scale and are thought by most physicists not to be applicable in domains larger than that of Plank's constant, that is photons and electrons, and that only traditional Newtonian mechanics applies to domains we experience in everyday life. Smith's (2003) proposal is that there is a hierarchical series of networks and domains in which quantum effects are transmitted to molecules through their vibrational energy states, and that molecules transfer this information to cells, and so forth, until the intact organism is involved, influenced and even engulfed by quantum effects.

Therefore, these results do not invalidate our "common-sense" materialism altogether. In the everyday world of "large" objects, the mechanistic causation of Newtonian physics is approximately correct, which is why much of medicine has been able to rely on it. However, contemporary Western medicine has not incorporated into its perspectives on health and healing these many clues and observations from fundamental science and contemporary physics about the nature of reality. Thus, Western society has advanced into the twenty-first century using cutting-edge technologies guided by nineteenth-century theories of materialist physics (and also typological biology). We can now look back on the formulations of ancient healers of Middle Asia in India, Tibet, and the Middle East, and understand how their "primitive" techniques can be interpreted in light of twenty-first-century physics, which will be demonstrated in the remainder of this book.

At the fundamental, subatomic level, materialism conflicts both with theory and with frequently replicated experimental evidence. This conflict gives rise to a fundamentally different worldview. Many physicists now argue that nature is composed of probability waves that are a function of intelligence or "consciousness" alone, not of discrete physical particles. The equations of quantum mechanics may ultimately be describing a world made of abstract patterns of intelligence.

In view of these uniformly idea-like characteristics of the quantum-physical world, the proper answer to the question, "What sort of world do we live in?" would seem to be: "We live in an idea-like world, not a matter-like world," as ultimately stated by Sir Arthur Eddington (1974)—who was knighted for his work. There is, in fact, in the quantum universe, no natural place for matter. This conclusion, curiously, is the exact reverse of the circumstance that in the classic physical universe there was not a natural place for mind and spirit.

In quantum field theory, the probability wave for a particle is described as a fluctuation in an underlying, nonmaterial field (known as a *force* field or matter *field*). Furthermore, in recent superunified theories, physicists have described all the force and matter fields that make up the universe as modes of vibration of one underlying, unified field, sometimes called the *superfield* or *superstring* field. All the order and intelligence of the laws of nature arise from this one fundamental, nonmaterial field, as does all matter. Not only are particles really just waves, but also those waves ultimately are made of an underlying field, as ocean waves are "made of" ocean water.

Intelligent life *is* the universe

This field is one of pure intelligence, having the attributes that we associate with consciousness. This field-effect lends support to the statement of the quantum mechanical pioneer Max Planck (1931), "I regard consciousness as fundamental. I regard matter as derivative from consciousness," and again, to Sir Arthur Eddington, the physicist who first provided evidence in support of Einstein's general theory of relativity, once derided by skeptics as Sir Arthur "Adding-One" who said, "The stuff of the world is mind-stuff" (Eddington 1974).

Unified field theory may seem worlds away from the concerns of medicine. The current Western or "allopathic" approach assumes that the body can be explained by material reductionism, analogous to machinery. Looking back through the lens of time at the ancient healing traditions of Middle Asia, in the light of modern physics, we may view the body as an abstract pattern of intelligence or information. Because this latter view appears to be consistent with fundamental science, it is reasonable to consider that it might contribute to the capacity to promote health. Contemporary efforts have been undertaken to understand the role of information in biology and the energetic information or imprint held in biological structures such as DNA.

While knowing nothing of DNA, and little of what modern science has established about the physical aspects of human anatomy, physiology, and biology—that is, *the human body*—the ancient healing traditions of Middle Asia were remarkably sophisticated regarding the perceptions of *body, mind and spirit* and how they interact to produce health and healing. That ancient information—as much wisdom as knowledge—can now be interpreted in light of what modern fundamental physics is telling us about the nature of reality itself.

Chapter 2

Vital Energy

Spirit and Flow

The idea of a "vital force" has been a core aspect of traditional healing practices for thousands of years in Middle Asia. In the West, this idea has been used to explain therapeutic practices such as Mesmerism, magnetic healing, and faith healing. The idea has also been part of discussions in Western science at least since 1907, when Henri Bergson proposed it as an explanation as to why organic molecules, the "chemicals of life," could *not* be synthesized (Bergson 1911). This thinking held that electricity—the physics and engineering wonder of the time— was somehow connected with this vital force. The contemporary expression of this idea is often called the biofield hypothesis (Rubik 2002). The important aspect of the biofield hypothesis is its dependence on classical electromagnetic fields and forces. Beverley Rubik, founder of the Center for Frontier Sciences in Philadelphia, now in San Francisco, states that the biofield is a useful construct consistent with bioelectromagnetics and the physics of nonlinear, dynamical, nonequilibrium living systems (Rubik 2002). Some aspects of vital healing may be explained with the biofield. It is completely consistent and even sufficient to explain magnetic therapy, for example. However, there are at least two aspects of some forms of energy healing that it does not adequately explain. One anomaly is the apparent *distance* independence. The other is the apparent instantaneous state change (like *quantum entanglement*) that is part of some forms of energy medicine. This second anomaly of energy healing is that it often happens *faster* than classical mechanisms can explain. It is possible that these anomalies, and the fundamental nature of vital healing, have their explanation in quantum physics. Others disagree, and still others feel that, although it is not the whole explanation, some aspects of quantum physics may be relevant and play a role in vital medicine (Dossey 2001).

If it is true that vital healing is often working through non-classical and quantum forms of energy, it is now possible to visualize a future where energy medicine uses a combination of classical forces and quantum energy fields to target and regulate endogenous processes and fields within the body to affect healing and well-being. If energy medicine and distant healing are fundamentally forms of information transfer, then quantum mechanics may provide the explanation and means for this process. It may explain not only the transfer of healing energy between people, but also the natural self-healing process itself. Rein (2004) has proposed that this information flow within the body is necessary for health, and that when it is impeded, ill-health and disease result. In this thinking, energy medicine is also the flow of information through quantum effects between healer and patient. In an analogous fashion, well-being and health are the free flow and transfer of information within the body, and the interchange of information with the environment to augment this flow. A new paradigm of understanding in medical science and health care may emerge that is as important and revolutionary as our biochemical models were in the twentieth century. But were some of these understandings from modern physics already being intuited by the ancient healers of Middle Asia, as well as the natural scientists and philosophers in the West who expanded their wonderment at Nature and human nature and began casting their gaze eastward in the seventeenth and eighteenth centuries?

The light of Asia

The period of Enlightenment in Europe came at the time of explorations throughout Asia and the Americas, and especially the settlement of the English colonies in "New England." At that time philosophical and scientific knowledge was broadly divided into Moral Philosophy (the laws of God) and Natural Philosophy (the laws of Nature), so that the aforementioned Sir Francis Bacon, for example, could safely practice both. All divisions in philosophy and knowledge are to some extent arbitrary, in terms of understanding ourselves and the universe. In the late twentieth century, the evolution of standard academic disciplines reveals more about academic careerism, tenure, and other tangential interests, than it continues to reveal truths about human nature and Nature.

Chapter 1 posited how to a considerable extent our deepest understandings of the universe are coming back into a "theory of everything," which had been Albert Einstein's ultimate quest, for example.

Already during the period of Colonial England and Early America, more unified perspectives were coming into contemplation. An important influence, even at that time, was knowledge from the exotic "Orient"—those regions that comprise the focus of this book—in Greater India and the Middle East. The introduction of Asian medicine to the West was not new to the twentieth century, but began to have a deliberate presence in Western thinking in the eighteenth and nineteenth centuries. Even then, when Europe was again emerging into the light, this knowledge and wisdom from Asia was already quite ancient.

Asian medical systems had an extensive history of texts, beliefs, and *materia medica* that had traversed mountains, steppes, plateaus, plains, deserts, and seas in circuits of exchange and trade. Medical systems flourished with the integration of medical theories, translations of texts, and practitioners contributing to various pedigrees of knowledge. These texts, practices, and pharmacopeia, shared across all these systems, reflect the following:

- The concept of disease as imbalance.

- The image of the body as a microcosm of the broader environment or as a reflection of cosmological order.

- An emphasis on dynamic vitality, often in terms of vital energy or energetic healing.

Vitality and its expression through energetic forms, such as the *prana* of Indian Ayurveda (much like the *qi* of Chinese medicine) provide a unifying theme in these Asian systems, which consider the body as an integral part of a broader universe of order and experience, and part of a greater whole that is connected by *energy* and *spirit*.

Further India, Greater China, and the influence of Islam

When considering the ancient medical traditions of India, Tibet, and the Middle East, it is useful to recognize all of South, East, and Southeast Asia as territories that came under the influence of two of the earliest civilizations at the dawn of history. The cultural diffusion concepts of "Further India" and "Greater China" are useful to consider as succeeding waves of influence emanating out from the great valleys of the Indus and the Yellow River, respectively, carrying along common discoveries and understandings of the nature of human life and health. Scholars of prehistoric humans locate the original center of Indian or Hindu culture and Sanskrit language texts in the Indus River Valley (modern-day Pakistan) in the second millennium BCE. These Indo-European (or Aryan) peoples, originally from the Caucusus Mountains, expanded east and south into the Indian subcontinent, establishing a new center in the Ganges River Valley, at the foot of the Himalayan Mountains, during the first millennium BCE, carrying the Sanskrit texts and knowledge with them. This Hindu civilization, which we associate with Ayurvedic medicine, and the related but separate practice of Yoga, pushed the Dravidian peoples, whom we associate with Siddha medicine, into the southeastern tip of India and onto the island of Ceylon, or Sri Lanka. One may see the subsequent outgrowth of Buddhism from the Hindu Prince Guatama (the

Buddha) as a manifestation of another wave of influence from "Further India" giving birth to the next waves in Tibet and Greater China.

Ultimately a third wave, Islam during the seven hundred years from 750 to 1450 CE, spread to the western border of North Africa, and to the eastern edge of Indonesia, carrying along Greek-Roman (*Unani*, Arabic for "Greek") concepts of health and healing, which it had incorporated and preserved following the Classical Era in the West. Bali, in the center of Indonesia, is a place which was substantially "skipped over" by Islam, and retained its Indian Vedic roots, while Sri Lanka, off the far southeast coast of India, and Timor, at the far eastern edge of Indonesia, represent fault lines which have had serious geopolitical repercussions into the twentieth century. All three of these great successive traditions placed emphasis on the concept of vital energy as central to health and healing.

East meets West

In India, in the geographic center of Asia, there were centuries of foreign rule, beginning in the fifteenth century, when invaders from Persia (modern-day Iran) occupied neighboring India, carrying the banner of Islam. They established the Mogul Empire, which was dominant especially in Northern India until the period of European colonization in Asia.

Initially, in the sixteenth century, the Portuguese established missions in South, Southeast, and East Asia under the dominions established by the Roman Catholic Pope by the Treaty of Tordesillas. This decree divided the globe into two hemispheres along a line of longitude through the Atlantic Ocean (and around the other side of the globe through the Pacific) between the "eastern" half, under Portuguese influence, and the "western" half, under Spanish influence, for purposes of trade and evangelization.

The borders of these "*hemispheres of influence*" extended around and over the globe such that the Portuguese had an outpost in Brazil in the New World at the western end of its eastern half of the world, while the Spanish developed a foothold in the Philippines in Asia at the far western end of its western half. India was firmly in the Portuguese half, as evidenced by the development of Goa, an active settlement of Portuguese Roman Catholic life to this day.

During the seventeenth century, the dominance of Portugal and Spain in global trade and colonization slowly gave way to the Dutch in South and Southeast Asia, and then during the eighteenth century to the French in India (Pondicherry) and Indochina, and to the English in India, Burma, and Malaya. During the nineteenth century, taking a hint from the Moguls, the British succeeed in establishing and organizing influence over the various princely states of India, culminating with the incoporation of India into the British Empire, adding the title "Empress of India" to Queen Victoria's reign. The Dutch focused their interests in the ancient territories of "Further India" in the Indonesian archipelago, where Bali still stands as a remnant of ancient Hindu and Vedic civilization among a sea of subsequent influences from China, Islam, and Europe.

Colonial England and early America

Influences from the ancient practice of medicine in Middle Asia date to the British colonial period, and early American history. These influences continued until their resurgence in late, or "postmodern," American and European history. Far from being just a recent import, Asian traditional cultural views of health and healing became very much part of what we consider to be American tradition. This early thinking and practice did not arise from physiologic or medical studies, but arose in the popular consciousness from non-medical cultural and spiritual movements based upon experiential and existential (not experimental) thinking, studies and philosophies. The abundance of Nature and the experience of "wilderness" to be found in America by the early English and European settlers gave early American thought a naturalistic bent, analogous to Asian perspectives on the health of the human body in relation to the natural environment and the cosmos. The tradition of meditative walking, especially in New England, was one means by which such thinking could come into practice, and a means by which such practices influenced uniquely American thinking.

In addition to the unique experience of the early American wilderness, meditative thought has antecedents inherited from European-Asian traditions brought to America. It is possible to date a European intellectual connection to Asian spiritual thought and practice as early as the ancient Greek histories of Herodotus, the Indian campaign of Alexander of Macedonia during 327–325 BCE, and Petrarch's mention of Hindu ascetics in his *Life of Solitude*, written 1345–1347 CE. Another beginning is the year 1784, the founding by British scholars and magistrates of the Asiatic Society of Bengal, from which quickly flowed the first translations of Hindu scriptures directly from Sanskrit texts into English.

Sir William Jones' translations of Kalidasa's *Sakuntala* (1789), Jayadeva's *Gitagovinda* (1792), and the *Institutes of Hindu Law* (1794) were influential. His early tutor in Sanskrit, Charles Wilkins, made the first translation of the *Bhagavad Gita* (1785). In 1788, the group founded a journal, *Asiatik Researches*, widely circulated among the intelligentsia, including second US president (1797–1801) and first resident of the White House, John Adams, and third president, Thomas Jefferson (1801–1809). Thus, one can imagine Hindu texts gracing the White House library and being incorporated into the new Library of Congress from Jefferson's founding collections from their earliest beginnings. This flow of scholarly and objective information about Indian culture and religion began a profound shift in Europe's and Early America's view of the East, from the earlier supposition of the East as barbarous and despotic, to a vision of an exotic and highly civilized world in its own right.

The new language, ideas, images, and narratives embedded in such texts immediately touched something in poets, philosophers, and artists in England, and were powerful influences on the development of American culture. The early-nineteenth-century Romantics in Europe embraced all things "Oriental" as a celebration of the irrational and exotic, in deliberate reaction to the prior Age of Reason, or Enlightenment. Their use of the scriptures, stories, lyrics, and images becoming ever more available to them from Hinduism, Buddhism, Confucianism, and Islam became an amalgam. However, their drive was not yet explicitly for a practical, "medical" use of these new elements of discourse in expressing some tacit knowledge heretofore inexpressible. Their Orientalism was not serious "science," but rather a matter of exotic settings for poems and literature, such as Samuel Taylor Coleridge's *Kublai Khan* (1798/1816):

> In Xanadu did Kubla Khan
> A stately pleasure dome decree;
> Where Alph, the sacred river, ran
> Through caverns measureless to man
> Down to a sunless sea

In North America, Edgar Allan Poe (1809–1849) picked up many of these themes in his pioneering literary works, such as *Tamerlane* (1827):

> Look round thee now on Samarcand!
> Is she not queen of Earth? Her pride
> Above all cities? In her hand
> Their destinies? In all beside...

These literary works carry images of the "oriental despotism" as well as the marvels, wonders, splendors and pleasures of the East. The subsequent confounding of international relations in the nineteenth and twentieth centuries by this Western romantic image of the Orient, or "Orientalism" (as in Edward Said's (1978) seminal work by the same name), was an unforeseen and serious consequence of carrying this image. The Romantics found "Oriental" thought a refreshing alternative to the stifling rationalism (and then nationalism) of their time. What they may have found in these explorations was the mind-energy-spirit which they associated with the "heart" rather than the "head"; since the seventeenth-century French philosopher and scientist Descartes had split the mind from the body in his philosophical discourses (in accommodation to the Church, although this criticism of him, and of the Church, is not entirely fair).

This appeal of Asian thought may have been based in the unity it brings to mind-body-spirit and its central role for a vital energy that animates both life and the universe. The concept of vital energy had not yet "given up the ghost," so to speak, in Europe at this time and could remain a preoccupation of late-eighteenth- and early-nineteenth-century scientists (for example, the Anglo-American—and Francophile—Benjamin Franklin, the French Antoine Lavoisier, and the German Alexander von Humboldt), while it was still possible to be both a moral and a natural philosopher.

Vital energy is central

While subsequently given up for a time in the science and medicine of the West, this concept of vital energy (*prana* in India, and *qi* in China) remained central to the Asian medical traditions, as it is to the modern reformulation of Maharishi Ayurveda, which consciously incorporates the insights of modern fundamental physics (while the ancient traditions appear to understand them implicitly).

In the meeting of East and West, *qi* has been translated to imply the flow of *energy, spirit, or breath* that animates living beings. Ancient Chinese ideograms depicted the term with three strokes to symbolize cloudlike vapor, as when the breath is seen on a cold day. In a more metabolic sense it may be seen as steam or vapor rising over rice or more generally, food. During the Song Dynasty in China (960–1127 CE), the term was elaborated to include four strokes (气), above the character for rice (米) and this form (氣) continues to be used in classical Chinese. Contemporary Chinese *pinyin* has simplified the term to the top four strokes (气), but without including the character beneath for rice. The character "vapor rising over rice" gives a more metabolic quality to this energy, versus what we might consider as electromagnetic energy or electricity. Further, the word "rice" (*fan*) has a more generic meaning as "food" or "foodstuff" as in the word *Fan-Djan* or "rice hall" meaning restaurant.

In the Chinese language, *qi* is ubiquitous, reflecting its wide usage in everyday contexts. It is a compound term having many meanings, and is used in words that describe a range of entities including atmosphere, environment, flavor, feeling, and emotional state. Thus context is crucial to understanding the influence of this *energy* in different forms.

Daoist texts, some as early as 300 BCE, with later recordings on bamboo wood and silk cloth, view *qi* as an elemental force that shapes both the universe as the human body and individual humans. *Qi* comes in many forms (from refined and immaterial to condensed and heavy). It can also be cultivated by the individual through breathing and special exercises (formulated as *qi gong*). Experiencing *qi*, and encounters with *qi*, can be quite subjective, but the overall view of *qi* as vital energy and regenerative force shows that health, life, and regeneration are not possible without it.

Healing unity

Asian medicine comprises multiple formulations of knowledge and practice within a broad range of ethnomedical traditions in the region. This chapter offers an overview of the knowledge and practice of *vital energy* common to these healing modalities and theories of the body. Within the specific context of medicine, the subjective and social experiences of *vital energy* come together. In Asian medical theory, *vital energy* takes on particular meaning, not simply as a force that stands alone, but as an entity that flows, interacts with the body-mind, and brings vital energy to the organs and channels (termed *meridians* in Chinese medicine, *chakras* in Indian Ayurveda) it traverses or inhabits. The cultivation of *vital energy* and its movement and flow—whether through meditation, yoga, or *qi gong*—is critical to well-being.

Asian medical history is rich with iconic texts, notable practitioners, and concepts that date back millennia. These medical systems are characterized as traditional, or unchanging, but have always had the ability to incorporate new concepts in continuity with the old. Kevin Ergil commented that, "Chinese medicine is a tradition that never threw anything away." It is important to recognize that each system of knowledge has significantly evolved—sometimes with the intervention of state institutions. Moreover, the diffusion of practitioners, translated texts, and herbal remedies and medicines across Asian medicine contributed to multiple forms and pedigrees of medical knowledge. The transmission of classic medical texts depended in part on regional proximity and cultural diffusion, as well as sharing the same written language, as was the case for Greater China, Japan, and Korea (where classical Chinese characters were used until the fifteenth century CE).

Another comparison considers the modalities or treatment techniques that may overlap or define distinct characteristics of a particular system. A third comparative framework is based upon regional ethnomedical practices utilizing *materia medica*, the use of plants with healing properties. Finally, we can observe the role of concepts such as vital energy through each of these approaches.

Vital energy, as *qi*, became integral for views of the body and medical practice in Asia at the origins of Chinese medicine and its later transmission to Korean and Japanese medicines. All three systems of Greater China refer to *qi* (*gi* or *ki*), as a form of energy that shapes all bodies. Vital energy is also important in *Ayurveda*, *Unani* (Greek-Islamic), and Tibetan medicines that bear resemblance to *qi* energy healing, and in the divine healing energy evident in Sufi healing practices.

The Spiritual Pivot

Classic texts in Chinese medicine date back to the second century BCE, and include sources ranging from silk documents excavated from the Mawangdui Han tombs (168 BCE, or earlier) to widely recorded works such as the *Huangdi Neijing* (黃帝 內經, *Yellow Emperor's "Inner Classic"* or *Canon of Internal Medicine*) and the *Shen Nong Bencaojing* (神農本草經, *Divine Husbandman's Materia Medica*). The latter is a compilation of plant and other medicinal substances and their influences on the body. The earliest mention of *qi* in the Mawangdui texts is in terms of vapor. Analysis of the Mawangdui texts suggests concepts of life nurturance and transformative practices were integrated with earlier ideas about *yangsheng* ("nurturing generation") through breath cultivation and meditation. These "evolving" categories preceded the more formal presentations of *qi* apparent in the later manuscripts of the *Huangdi Neijing*.

The *Huangdi Neijing* consists of two texts (the *Suwen*, 素問, or "Basic Questions" and *Lingshu*, 靈樞, "Spiritual Pivot"). The chapters are composed as a dialogue or series of questions and answers between the Yellow Emperor, *Huangdi*, and his ministers, such as *Qi Bo*. *Suwen* and its various translations address the role of *qi* as foundational to the body, and the term is often used together with Blood (*xue*, 血). Where *qi* flows so goes Blood. Considerable discussion is devoted to the Five Organs (*zang*, 臟)—the Heart (*xin*, 心), Spleen (*pi*, 脾), Lung (*fei*, 肺), Kidney (*shen*, 腎), and Liver (*gan*, 肝)—and how each of these organs harbor different forms of *qi*. This correspondence is also referred to as the Five Phases (*wuxing*, 五行). The Organs not only house but also facilitate relations between *qi* and various emotional states:

> When one is angry, the *qi* rises.
> When one is happy, the *qi* is relaxed.
> When one is sad, then the *qi* dissipates.
> When one is in fear, then the *qi* moves down.

Qi is a multivalent term used to refer not only to vapor but also to a range of bodily states and transformations due to disorder and disease. Movement of *qi* determines health, while the cessation of this movement, or stagnation, means disease or ultimately death. Circulation is crucial—as suggested by the correlation of bodily channels and organs to government ministerial posts and functions, which indicate intimate correspondences among body, cosmos, and state. The flow of *qi* within bodily structures guided both political structures and rightful rule, with the greater order in the cosmos reflected in ancient Chinese bureaucracy.

The original text of the *Lingshu*, the second part of the *Huangdi Neijing*, no longer exists, and translations are based on later editions from the twelfth century. The *Lingshu* (*Spiritual Pivot*) is also called the *Canon or "Classic" of Acupuncture*, and mainly addresses the meridians (*jingluo*, 經絡) or pathways for the circulation of *qi*, and the acupuncture points (*zhenxue*, 針穴), through which *qi* enters and leaves the body. *Qi* remains the central concept, as its flow, or movement within the body, can be influenced by acupuncture techniques.

These classical texts trace the concept of *qi* and demonstrate how it became integral to theories about the human body and medical treatment. These concepts diffused with the transmission of medicine took hold where exchange occurred across and beyond Greater China. Both Korean and Japanese medicine utilize the concept of *gi* or *ki* based on early translations of Chinese medical texts and the introduction of Chinese medical practitioners to their royal courts.

Adoption of Chinese medical theory and *materia medica* took place sooner in Korea, in light of its more proximal location within Greater China. Medical texts such as the *Suwen* were exported to Korea during China's Song Dynasty (970–1279). Early forms of Korean medicine utilized Chinese medical theories of *yin* (陰) and *yang* (陽) (the opposite but complementary qualities of all things), meridians, acupuncture, and *qi*. Later forms of Korean medicine evolved, with the incorporation of herbal remedies indigenous to the area, and with the arrival of charismatic Buddhist monks focused on healing. Eventually a hybrid system of knowledge, utilizing Chinese medical concepts and local plants, became a foundation of traditional Korean medicine. As with Chinese medicine, prominent doctors promulgated their techniques and writings regarding medical beliefs and practices.

During the fifth and sixth centuries, Chinese medicine was also introduced to Japan by travelers between the two countries, including court emissaries, physicians and Buddhist monks. The Song Dynasty medical source texts also facilitated this transmission of knowledge. As with Korea, the Japanese integration of Chinese medicine incorporated basic medical principles of *ki*, and *yin–yang* notions of balance. Premodern Japanese medical texts such as the *Ishimpo* (*Methods at the Heart of Medicine*) and Menase Dosan's sixteenth-century multivolume medical writings utilize these Chinese medical theories in their discussion of diseases and treatments. Japanese medicine was also influenced by the practice of Zen and other forms of Buddhism. From the late eighteenth century, it was influenced as well by Western medical knowledge introduced by the Dutch. Traditional Japanese medicine developed specialized knowledge of acupressure (*shiatsu*), and distinct techniques in acupuncture, bone manipulation and setting techniques.

Kampo (漢方), the contemporary form of Chinese medicine in Japan, has integrated evidence-based research and biomedical theory. *Ki* is now described as a vital energy that allows the mind and body to function appropriately, may correspond to activities of the central nervous system (CNS) and autonomic nervous system, and can be disturbed by psychosocial stressors.

The diffusion of Chinese medicine to other regions in Asia went by many paths to healing. Official state delegations, medicinal herb traders, spiritual pilgrims, and itinerant healers spread Chinese medicine and throughout the Asia of Greater China. The presence of Chinese medicine persists to this day across Greater China, present-day Southeast Asia, Central Asia, and South Asia. The concept of *qi*, its cultivation, and flow, as well as the meridians or channels in which *qi* flows, or can be blocked or become stagnant, are key considerations for pathology and therapeutics, and unifies the different systems.

Flowing on the Silk Road

As traders, nomads, and emissaries traversed the Silk Road, Chinese medical texts and medicinal herbs were carried along. Chinese medicine and concepts of *qi* reached the Southern and Central Asian regions where traditional medicines with their own ideas of energetic healing were already being practiced, such as Ayurveda, Unani, and Tibetan medicine. The flow of energy within a body as a source of vitality is a concept shared by nearly all Asian medical systems. Indigenous ethnomedicine, based on local knowledge of plants and herbs, allowed the establishment of local, vital forms of medical practice.

Vital energy in South Asia

Ayurveda emerged in South Asia, and is considered to have a history of nearly five thousand years. Translated as the "knowledge or science of life," this system of healing consists of a range of practices including meditation, *yoga*, massage, diet, and herbal medicines and tonics. Galenic medicine from ancient Rome and Greece, and its belief in humors, closely parallel Ayurveda. Human bodies are constituted by three, rather than four, main humoral entities, or *doshas*: *pitta* (bile), *vata* (wind), and *kapha* (phlegm). Another central concept is *prana*, considered to be the "breath of life," and thus analogous to the concept of *qi*. It is part of a trilogy of forces, including *agni* (the spirit of light or fire) and *soma* (harmony and love). The Hindu texts from the first millennium, the Upanishads, are among the first to refer to *prana* as part of the physical world, providing the vital energy that sustains all living forms. The later philosophies that form the basis of *yoga* consider *prana* to flow through subtle channels (*nadi*, "tubes") in the body, through which pass bodily fluids—as with blood and *qi*, as well as semen. In Ayurvedic thought, *prana* is further differentiated into five forms, known as the *prana vayu*, which sustain bodily processes, such as circulation (*prana*), digestion (*samana*), elimination (*apana*), vocalizing sounds (*udana*), and movement (*vyana*).

Like *qi gong*, or cultivation of *qi* (which also have five forms) in Chinese medicine, *pranayama* in India is the practice of attaining and cultivating *prana*, initially through breathwork and breath control techniques. The similarities, and differences, between *qi* and *prana* have been much debated by scholars of Asian medicine and spiritual practices. Similarity has been noted between the practices of hatha yoga and *daoyin* (導引), considered to be the precursor of most forms of *qi gong*. However, *yoga* and *qi gong* are not the same. These practices reflect comparable developments in concepts of self-cultivation and transformation since the thirteenth century (see Chapter 5).

To the High Himalaya

As with other Asian medical systems, Tibetan medicine evolved in the presence of ideas and materials exchanged over the Himalayan Mountains, through trade and traveling practitioners. Regional exchanges along the Silk Road and collaboration between foreign scholars in Tibet between the eighth and eleventh centuries were extensive. Tibetan medicine incorporated theories from multiple sources of knowledge, including Ayurvedic, Persian, ancient Greek, Central Asian, and Chinese medicine. Ayurvedic medicine influenced this system, but Tibetan concepts of the body are more complex, and even convoluted, with up to fifteen subcategories of humors, while also incorporating the ideas of *karma* and Buddhist philosophy. More than other Asian medical systems, Tibetan medicine consciously joins medical knowledge with the traditions of Buddhism, particularly, ideals of compassion and activity in the service of others.

While Chinese medicine describes up to five types of *qi*, Tibetan medicine conceptualizes the body as based on three vital *ñes-pa*, which in turn can be seen as similar to the Ayurvedic *doshas*, or constitutional types. The Tibetan types are *rLung*, wind (cold, subtle, volatile), *mKhris-pa*, bile (hot, liquid, flowing), and *Bad-kan*, phlegm (cool, sluggish, solid). There are seven principal bodily constituents (saliva, blood, bone, marrow, flesh, fat, and semen). Of the *ñes-pa*, the nearest to *qi* is *rLung*. Careful attention is accorded to the breath, as every living entity is animated by the "breath of life" or *spirit*.

Theories of causation reflect close correspondence with Buddhist beliefs about physical, emotional, and mental states. Initial clinical diagnosis may include pulse reading, observation, inquiry, and urine analysis. The therapeutic modalities depend upon the severity of symptoms, and include golden needle treatment, moxibustion, medicinal baths, enemas, purgatives, or massage, in combination with spiritual prayer, Five Element color therapy, and astrological consultation. There are definite overlaps with Ayurvedic and Chinese medicine, but Tibetan medicine has evolved over the centuries to form a distinctive body of medical knowledge and views of the body.

It's all Greek, too

Another medical system originating in the ancient world was Greek medicine, whose texts were later translated by Persian scholars during the Islamic period. Its influence can be seen today in Unani medicine which, like Ayurveda, is practiced mostly in South Asia. Unani means "Greek" and refers to the pedigree of Greco-Islamic medical knowledge, which can be traced through the treatises of Avicenna (Ibn Sina) and Galen, back to Hippocrates in the fifth century BCE. During the thirteenth to seventeenth centuries, Unani practitioners from Persia and Central Asia enjoyed special patronage from the Persian Mogul (Islamic) courts as well as from Indian elites.

Unani overlaps significantly with Ayurvedic principles. Both systems rely on the concept of the humors, which shape human bodies and temperaments, and on the concept of vital energy, which is central to life (*pneuma* in Greek) or spirit. Although there are some similarities and correspondences in concepts of bodily constitution and vital energy, as well as herbal formularies, Unani differs in several origins. Ayurvedic texts are mostly derived from Sanskrit and Hindu sources, while Unani manuscripts are mainly from Arabic and Persian texts. Another difference is in the preparation of plant remedies, including spices and herbs. Unani relies on the classic Greek theory of four humors and their balance which can be obtained from fluids. Unani preferentially uses herbal tonics based on old recipes for syrups (as well as powders, pills, and tablets). These remedies are still manufactured and sold to a broad consumer base, including younger generations, in urban India.

Like Chinese and Tibetan medicine, Unani uses pulse diagnosis and examination of the tongue, urine, and stool to evaluate sources of imbalance. Corresponding with Chinese medicine, therapeutic modalities also include cupping, sweating, diuresis, bathing, massage, cauterization, purging, and leeching (bleeding). Diet therapy tends to be used in preference to pharmaceuticals, while surgery is reserved as only the last resort.

In addition to the Greco-Arabic Unani (also in Arabic, *Tibb*) medical system, translated and carried forward to this day by Islam, Islam also developed a more purely spiritual, or devotional, form of healing through Sufi mysticism. While Tibetan medicine is the form of Middle Asian medicine most consonant with Buddhism, Sufi healing is the form most consonant with Islam, and, indeed, forms an expression of Islamic devotion, just as the traditional purpose of Yoga in India is also devotional. Sufi healing, while having many guidelines having to do with care of the body, is perhaps mostly purely a manifestation of spirit among these healing traditions. The route to health and, more broadly, enlightenment and healthy life ways, is through the body to the spirit—as in Hatha Yoga, for example.

In the midst of the age-old struggle to keep body and spirit together in Asian societies, they developed means for seeking the one through the other in vital and dynamic ways, as well as contemplative and meditative means, whether Ayurveda, Siddha, Unani or Sufi.

The following chapters further explore the *energy* and *spirit* of each of these many traditional paths for health and healing in the Middle Asia of Further India, Greater China and the sphere of Islam.

Chapter 3

Continuous Healing

Traditional Ayurvedic Medicine

Three traditional Middle Asian medicinal systems predominate in modern India: Ayurveda, Siddha, and Unani. Ayurveda is found mostly in Northern India and in Kerala in the south. Siddha medicine is found mostly in Tamil Nadu and in parts of Kerala (see Chapter 4). Unani is found throughout India and Pakistan, mainly in the urban areas, and actually derives from Arabic medicine, rather than Indian sources (see Chapter 8). This chapter describes Ayurveda, and following chapters discuss the other, related traditional systems, Siddha medicine (see Chapter 4), yoga (see Chapter 5), and the contemporary development of Maharishi Ayurveda in India and the West (see Chapter 6). Traditional medicine, in addition to being a highly developed and complex form of "ethnomedicine," remains in living use as an available form of primary health care in India; as well it is becoming more available in the West as a "complementary/alternative" medical system that is accessed in the practice of "integrative medicine."

The science of life

Ayurveda is, literally, the science of life, or longevity. As with any popular development, aspects of this Indian medical system and its cures have sometimes been appropriated by individuals not wholly familiar with the basic assumptions of Ayurveda as a science of longevity. However, scholars have undertaken serious study of this ancient healing tradition. The fundamental principles and practices of traditional Ayurveda may be understood from their work on the classical Sanskrit sources and from accounts from traditional Indian practitioners.

Four phases

On the basis of available literary sources, the history of Indian medicine occurred in four main phases (Zysk 1991, 1993). The first, or Vedic, phase dates from about 1200 to 800 BCE. Information about medicine during this period is obtained from numerous curative incantations and references to healing that are found in the *Atharvaveda* and the *Rigveda*, two religious scriptures that reveal a "magico-religious" approach to healing (Zysk 1993). The second, or classical, phase is marked by the advent of the first Sanskrit medical treatises, the *Caraka Samhita* (Sharma 1981–1994) and *Sushruta Samhita* (Bhishagratna 1983), which probably date from a few centuries before to several centuries after the start of the common era. This period includes all medical treatises dating from before the Muslim invasions of India at the beginning of the eleventh century. These works tend to follow the earlier classical compilations closely, and provide the basis of traditional Ayurveda. The third, or syncretic, phase is marked by clear influences from Unani, Siddha, and other non-classical medical systems in India. Bhavamishra's sixteenth century *Bhavaprakasha* is one text that reveals the results of these influences, such as diagnosis by examination of pulse or urine (Upadhyay 1986). This phase extends from the time of the Muslim incursions to the present era. I have phrased the fourth phase as "New Age Ayurveda," wherein the classical paradigm is being adapted to the world of modern science and technology, including quantum physics, mind-body science, and advanced biomedical science. This recent manifestation of Ayurveda is most visible in the Western world, although there are indications that it is filtering back to India in its worldwide reach (see Chapter 6). These four phases of Indian medical history provide a chronological grid for understanding the development of this ancient system of medicine (see Table 3.1).

Table 3.1 Phases of Ayurvedic medicine

Phase	Dates	Sources	Modalities
I. Vedic	1200–800 BCE	*Atharvaveda,* *Rigveda*	Magico-religious
II. Classic	700 BCE–400 CE	Sanskrit texts *Caraka,* *Sushruta,* *Samhita*	Herbal medicines
III. Syncretic	1000–1980 CE	Muslim influences, Unani, Siddha *Bhavaprakasha*	Pulse, urine diagnosis
IV. New Age	1980–2010 CE	Maharishi Ayurveda	Quantum physics

From its beginnings during the Vedic era, Indian medicine has always adhered closely to the principle of a fundamental connection between the microcosm and macrocosm. Human beings are minute representations of the universe, and contain within them everything that makes up the surrounding world. Comprehending the world is crucial to comprehending the human, and, conversely, understanding the world is necessary to understanding the human.

The five elements

According to Ayurveda, the cosmos consists of five basic elements: earth, air, fire, water, and space. Certain forces cause these to interact, giving rise to all that exists. In human beings these five elements occur as the three *doshas*, forces that, along with the seven *dhatus* (tissues) and three *malas* (waste products), make up the human body.

The three doshas

When in equilibrium the three doshas maintain health, but when an imbalance occurs among them, they defile the normal functioning of the body, leading to the manifestation of disease. An imbalance indicates an increase or decrease in one, two, or all three of the doshas. The three doshas are *vata*, *pitta*, and *kapha* (Svoboda 1984).

Vata or *vayu*, meaning "wind," is composed of the elements air and space. It is the principle of kinetic energy and is responsible for all bodily movement and nervous functions. It is located below the navel, in the bladder, large intestines, nervous system, pelvic region, thighs, bone marrow, and legs; its principal seat is the colon. When disrupted, its primary manifestations are gas and muscular or nervous energy, leading to pain.

Pitta or bile is made up of the elements fire and water. It governs enzymes and hormones, and is responsible for digestion, pigmentation, body temperature, hunger, thirst, sight, courage, and mental activity. It is located between the navel and the chest, in the stomach, small intestines, liver, spleen, skin, and blood; its principal seat is the stomach. When disrupted, its primary manifestations are acid and bile, leading to inflammation.

Kapha, meaning "phlegm," is made up of the elements of earth and water. It connotes the principle of cohesion and stability. It regulates vata and pitta and is responsible for keeping the body lubricated, and maintaining its solid nature, tissues, sexual power, and strength. It also controls patience. Its normal locations are the upper part of the body, the thorax, head, neck, upper portion of the stomach, pleural cavity, fat tissues, and areas between joints; its principal seat is the lungs. When it is disrupted, its primary manifestations are liquid and mucus, leading to swelling, with or without discharge.

The attributes of each dosha help determine an individual's basic bodily and mental makeup and to isolate which dosha is responsible for a disease. *Vata* is dry, cold, light, irregular, mobile, rough, and abundant. Dryness occurs when vata is disturbed, and is a side effect of motion. Too much dryness produces irregularity in the body and mind. *Pitta* is hot, light, intense, fluid, liquid, putrid, pungent, and sour. Heat appears when pitta is disturbed, and produces irritability in the body and mind. *Kapha* is heavy, unctuous, cold, stable, dense, soft, and smooth. Heaviness occurs when kapha is disturbed, and produces slowness in body and mind.

The seven dhatus

The seven *dhatus*, or tissues, are responsible for sustaining the body. Each dhatu is responsible for the one that comes next in the following order, according to Zysk:

1. *Rasa*, meaning sap or juice, includes the tissue fluids, bile, lymph, and plasma, and functions as nourishment. It comes from digested food.

2. Blood includes the red blood cells and functions to invigorate the body.

3. Flesh includes muscle tissue and functions as stabilization.

4. Fat includes adipose tissue and functions as lubrication.

5. Bone includes bone and cartilage and functions as support.

6. Marrow includes red and yellow bone marrow and functions as filling for the bones.

7. *Shukra* includes male and female sexual fluids and functions in reproduction and immunity.

(Zysk 1993)

The three malas

The *malas* are the waste products of digestion. Ayurveda delineates three principal malas: urine, feces, and sweat. A fourth category of other waste products includes fatty excretions from the skin and intestines, cebum (ear wax), mucus of the nose, saliva, tears, hair, and nails. According to Ayurveda, an individual should evacuate the bowels once a day and eliminate urine six times a day.

The importance of digestion

Ayurveda considers digestion to be the most important function that takes place in the human body. It provides all that is required to sustain the organism and is the principal cause for all maladies from which an individual suffers. The process of digestion and assimilation of nutrients is discussed under the topics of the *agnis* (enzymes), *ama* (improperly digested food and drink), and the *srotas* (channels of circulation).

The three agnis

The agnis, or enzymes, assist in the digestion and assimilation of food and are divided into three types, according to Zysk:

1. *Jatharagni* is active in the mouth, stomach, and gastrointestinal tract and helps break down food. The waste product of feces results from this activity.

2. *Bhutagnis* are five enzymes located in the liver. They adapt the broken down food into a homologous chyle in accordance with the five elements, and assist the chyle to assimilate with the corresponding elements in the body. The homologous chyle circulates in the blood channels as rasa, nourishing the body and supplying the seven dhatus.

3. *Dhatvagnis* are seven enzymes that synthesize the seven dhatus from the assimilated chyle homologized with the five elements. The remaining waste products result from this activity.

(Zysk 1993)

Ama

Ama is the chief cause of disease and is formed when there is a decrease in enzyme activity. A product of improperly digested food and drink, it takes the form of a liquid sludge that travels through the same channels as the chyle. Because of its density, however, it lodges in different parts of the body, blocking the channels. It often mixes with the doshas that circulate through the same pathways, and it gravitates to a weak or stressed organ or to a site of a disease manifestation. Because all diseases invariably come from ama, the word *amaya*, meaning "coming from ama," is a synonym for disease. Internal diseases begin with ama, and external diseases produce ama. In general, ama can be detected by a coating on the tongue; turbid urine with foul odor; and feces that is passed with undigested food, an offensive odor, and abundant gas. The principal course of treatment in Ayurveda involves the elimination of ama and the restoration of the balance of the doshas.

The thirteen kinds of srotas

The srotas are the vessels or channels of the body through which all substances circulate. They are either large, such as the large and small intestines, uterus, arteries, and veins, or small, such as the capillaries. A healthy body has open and free-flowing channels. Blockage of the channels, usually by ama, results in disease (Zysk 1993).

1. *Pranavahasrotas* convey vitality and vital breath (*prana*), and originate in the heart and alimentary tract.

2. *Udakavahasrotas* convey water and fluids, and originate in the palate and pancreas.

3. *Annavahasrotas* convey food from the outside, and originate in the stomach.

4. *Rasavahasrotas* convey chyle, lymph, and plasma, and originate in the heart and in the ten vessels connected with the heart. Ama primarily accumulates within them.

5. *Raktavahasrotas* convey red blood cells, and originate in the liver and spleen.

6. *Mamsavahasrotas* convey ingredients for muscle tissue, and originate in the tendons, ligaments, and skin.

7. *Medovahasrotas* convey ingredients for fat tissue, and originate in the kidneys and fat tissues of the abdomen.

8. *Asthavahasrotas* convey ingredients for bone tissue, and originate in hip bone.

9. *Majjavahasrotas* convey ingredients for marrow, and originate in the bones and joints.

10. *Shukravahasrotas* convey ingredients for the male and female reproductive tissues, and originate in the testicles and ovaries.

11. *Mutravahasrotas* convey urine, and originate in the kidney and bladder.

12. *Purishavahasrotas* convey feces, and originate in the colon and rectum.

13. *Svedavahasrotas* convey sweat, and originate in the fat tissues and hair follicles.

(Zysk 1993)

Constitutional types

This broad outline presents the Ayurvedic view that the human body's anatomical parts are composed of the five basic elements, which have undergone a process of metabolism and assimilation in the body. Human beings differ in their normal bodily constitution (*prakriti*), which is determined at the moment of conception, and remains so until death. The four factors that influence constitutional type include the father, the mother (particularly her food intake), the womb, and the season of the year. A large imbalance of the doshas in the mother will affect the growth of the embryo and fetus, and a moderate excess of one or two of the doshas will affect the constitution of the child.

Prakriti

There are seven normal body constitutions (*prakriti*) based on the three doshas: *vata, pitta, kapha, vata-pitta, pitta-kapha, vata-kapha,* and *sama*. The last is triple balanced, which is best, but extremely rare. Most people are a combination of doshas, in which one dosha predominates. In general, vata-type people tend to be anxious and fearful, exhibit light and "airy" characteristics, and are prone to vata-diseases. Pitta-type people are aggressive and impatient, exhibit fiery and hot-headed characteristics, and are prone to pitta-diseases. Kapha-type people are stable and entrenched, exhibit heavy, wet, and earthy characteristics, and are prone to kapha-diseases (Svoboda 1984).

These are the principal factors that help guide the Ayurvedic physician to determine the correct course of treatment to be administered to a patient for a particular ailment.

Mental states

In addition to physical constitution, Ayurveda understands that an individual is influenced by three mental states, based on the three qualities (*gunas*) of balance (*sattva*), energy (*rajas*), and inertia (*tamas*). In the state of balance the mind is in equilibrium and can discriminate correctly. In the state of energy the mind is excessively active, causing weakness in discrimination. In the state of inertia the mind is excessively inactive, also creating weak discrimination.

Ayurveda always has recognized that the body and the mind interact to create a healthy, normal (*prakriti*) or unhealthy, abnormal (*vikriti*) condition. A good Ayurvedic physician will determine both the mental and physical condition of the patient before proceeding with any form of diagnosis and treatment.

The naming of disease

Aspects of the Ayurvedic understanding of disease have been mentioned above. These understandings provide a basis for the Ayurvedic classification of disease, the naming of disease, and the manifestations of disease (Dash 1980; Dash and Kashyap 1980).

Ayurveda identifies three broad categories of disease, on the basis of causative factors:

1. *Adhyatmika* diseases originate within the body, and may be subdivided into hereditary diseases, congenital

diseases, and diseases caused by one or a combination of the doshas.

2. *Adhibhautika* diseases originate outside the body, and include injuries from accidents or mishaps, and, in the terminology of the modern era, from germs, viruses, and bacteria.

3. *Adhidaivika* diseases originate from supernatural sources, including diseases that are otherwise inexplicable, such as maladies stemming from providential causes, planetary influences, curses, and seasonal changes.

(Zysk 1993)

A six-step process that determines the manner by which a dosha becomes aggravated and moves through the different channels to produce disease. An accumulation of a dosha leads to its aggravation, which causes it to spread through the channels until it lodges in a particular organ of the body, bringing about a manifestation of disease. Once a general form of the disease appears, it progressively divides into specific varieties. As in systems of medicine worldwide, many patients consult the Ayurvedic physician only after the disease appears.

Ayurveda delineates seven basic varieties of disease on the basis of the doshas: diseases involving a single dosha, diseases involving two doshas, and diseases involving all three doshas together.

In Ayurveda, diseases receive their names in one of six ways. A disease is named for the condition it produces (fever, or *Jvara*), its chief symptom (diarrhea, or *Atisara*), its chief physical sign (jaundice, or *Pandu*), its principal nature (piles, or *Arshas*), the chief dosha(s) involved (wind-disease, or *Vata-roga*), or the chief organ involved (disease of the duodenum, or *Grahani*). Regardless of its given name, most diseases are understood to involve one or more of the doshas.

During the course of a disease an Ayurvedic physician seeks to identify its site of origin, its path of transportation, and its site of manifestation. The site of manifestation of a disease usually differs from its site of origin. Recognizing this distinction enables the physician to determine the correct course of treatment.

> Ayurveda describes the manifestation of all diseases in the same fundamental way. Causative factors (e.g., food, drink, regimen, season, mental state) suppress digestive (enzyme) activity in the body, leading to the formation of ama. The circulating ama blocks the channels. The site of the disease's origin is where the blockage occurs. The circulating ama, often combining with one or more of the doshas, then takes a divergent course, referred to as the *path of transportation*. Finally, the dosha(s) and ama mixture comes to rest in and afflicts a certain body part, which is known as the *site of disease manifestation*. Treatment entails correction of all the steps in the process resulting in disease manifestation, thus restoring the entire person to his or her particular balanced state. (Zysk 1993)

Diagnosis and treatment

In Ayurveda restoring a person to health is not viewed simply as the eradication of disease. It entails a complete process of diagnosis and therapeutics that takes into account both mental and physical components integrated with the social and physical worlds in which the patient lives. It begins with Ayurvedic diagnosis, examination of the disease, and types of therapeutics (Jolly 1977; Lad 1990; Sen Gupta 1984).

Ayurveda uses a detailed system of diagnosis, involving examination of pulse, urine, and physical features. After a preliminary examination by means of visual observation, touch, and interrogation, the Ayurvedic physician undertakes an eightfold method of detailed examination to determine the patient's type of physical constitution and mental status and to get an indication of any abnormality.

Feeling the pulse: snakes, frogs, and birds

The first mention of pulse examination is in a medical treatise from the late thirteenth to early fourteenth centuries of the common era. It is a highly specialized art and not every Ayurvedic physician uses pulse examination. The diagnostic process involves evenly placing the index, middle, and ring fingers of the right hand on the radial artery of the right hand of men and the left hand of women, just at the base of the thumb. A pulse resembling the movement of a snake at the index finger indicates a predominance of vata; a pulse resembling the movement of a frog at the middle finger indicates a predominance of pitta; a pulse resembling the movement of a swan or peacock at the ring finger indicates a predominance of kapha; and a pulse resembling the pecking of a woodpecker in all three fingers indicates a predominance of all three doshas. To get an accurate reading, the physician must keep in mind the times when each of the doshas are normally excited, and should take the pulse at least three times, making sure to wash his or her hands after each reading. Optimum timing for the reading is early in the morning when the stomach is empty, or three hours after eating in the afternoon (Upadhyay 1986).

Urine examination: the shapes of drops

Like pulse examination, urine examination probably was formalized in the syncretic phase (see Table 3.1). After collecting a midstream urine evacuation in a clear glass container, after sunrise the physician submits the urine to two kinds of examination. First, the physician studies it in the container to determine its color and degree of transparency. Pale yellow and oily urine indicates vata; intense yellow, reddish, or blue urine indicates pitta; white, foamy, and muddy urine indicates kapha; urine with a blackish tinge indicates a combination of doshas; and urine resembling lime juice or vinegar indicates ama. The physician also puts a few drops of sesame oil in the urine and examines it in sunlight. The shape, movement, and diffusion of the oil in the urine indicate the prognosis of the disease. The shape of the drops also reveals which dosha(s) is involved. A snakelike shape indicates vata; umbrella shape, pitta; and pearl shape, kapha.

Examining the body

The physician concludes the diagnostic examination with careful scrutiny of the tongue, skin, nails, and physical features to determine which dosha(s) is affected. Using the basic characteristics of each of the doshas, the physician will examine the different parts of the body. Coldness, dryness, roughness, and cracking indicate vata; hotness and redness indicate pitta; and wetness, whiteness, and coldness indicate kapha.

Having completed this phase of the diagnosis, the Ayurvedic physician proceeds to examine any malady present.

Five steps

A detailed examination of the disease involves a *five-step process*, leading to a complete understanding of the abnormality (Zysk 1993).

1. *Finding the cause*: a disease is *caused* by one or several of the following factors: mental imbalances resulting from the effects of past actions (*karma*); unbalanced contact between the senses and the objects of the senses affecting the body and the mind; effects of the seasons on the mental and doshic balance; the immediate causes of diet, regimen, and micro-organisms; doshas and ama; and the interaction of individual components such as doshas and tissues or doshas and micro-organisms.

2. *Early signs and symptoms*: signs and symptoms appear before the onset of disease and provide clues to the diagnosis. Proper diet and administration of medicine can avert disease if it is recognized early enough.

3. *Manifest signs and symptoms*: the most crucial step in the diagnostic process involves determining the site of origin, site of disease manifestation, and the path of transportation of the ama and dosha(s). Most signs and symptoms are associated with the site of manifestation, from which the physician must work his or her way back to the site of origin to effect a complete cure. Although symptomatic treatment was largely absent in traditional Ayurveda, modern medicine in India

has introduced Ayurvedic physicians to techniques of symptomatic treatment in cases of acute disease.

4. *Exploratory therapy*: this empirical step involves 18 different experiments that use herbs, diet, and regimens to determine the precise nature of the malady and suitable therapy by allopathic and homeopathic ("proving") means.

5. *Prognosis*: because Ayurvedic physicians traditionally did not treat persons with incurable diseases, it was important for the physician to know precisely the patient's chances of recovery. Therefore, a disease is classified as one of three types. It is easily curable, palliative, or incurable or difficult to cure.

While working with Trudy van Houten at the Museum Applied Science Center for Archaeology, University of Pennsylvania Museum, Philadelphia during 1981, the author noted the following in translations of the ancient Egyptian medical document known as the Edwin Smith Papyrus (named after the Victorian gentleman who originally acquired it from Egypt): diseases of the head and neck are categorized as "diseases I will treat," implying the expectation of cure, "diseases with which I will contend," implying the expectation to alleviate suffering, and "diseases I will not treat," implying the incurable. In general, if the disease type (vata, pitta, kapha) is different from the person's normal physical constitution, the disease is easy to cure. If the disease and constitution are the same, the disease is difficult to cure. If the disease, constitution, and season correspond to doshic type, the disease is nearly impossible to cure.

Having determined the patient's normal constitution, diagnosed his or her illness, and established a prognosis for recovery, the Ayurvedic physician can begin a proper course of treatment.

Continuous healing

Ayurveda recognizes two courses of treatment on the basis of the condition of the patient. The first is prevention, for the healthy person who wants to maintain a normal condition based on his or her physical constitution and to prevent disease. The second is therapy, for an ill person who requires health to be restored. Once healthy, Ayurveda recommends continuous prophylaxis based on diet, regimen, medicines, and regular therapeutic purification procedures.

When a person is diagnosed with a doshic imbalance, either purification therapy, alleviation therapy, or a combination of these is prescribed.

Purification: the five actions

Purification therapy involves the fundamental five actions, or *Panchakarma*, treatment. This fivefold process varies slightly in different traditions and regions of India, but a standard regimen generally is followed. All five procedures can be performed, or a selection of procedures can be chosen on the basis of different factors such as the physical constitution of the patient, his or her condition, the season, and the nature of the disease.

1. Before any action is taken, the patient is given oil internally and externally (with massage) and is sweated to loosen and soften the dosha(s) and ama.

2. An appropriate diet of food and drink is prescribed.

After this two-part preparatory treatment, called *Purvakarma*, the five therapies are administered in sequence over the period of about a week.

The patient is advised to set aside time for treatment in light of the profound effects on the mind and body. First, the patient might be given an emetic to induce vomiting until bilious matter is produced, thus removing kapha. Second, a purgative is given until mucus material appears, thus removing pitta. Third, an enema, either of oil or decocted medicines, is administered, flushing the bowels, to remove excess vata. Fourth, head purgation is given in the form of smoke inhalation or nasal drops to eradicate the dosha(s) that have accumulated in the head and sinuses. Fifth, leeches may be applied and bloodletting performed to purify the blood. Some physicians do not consider bloodletting in the five therapies of *Panchakarma*, instead counting oily and dry (decocted medicine) enemas as two separate forms (Singh 1992).

Alleviation: basic condiments

Alleviation therapy uses the basic condiments honey, butter or ghee, and sesame oil or castor oil to eliminate kapha, pitta, and vata, respectively. This therapy and *Panchakarma* are often employed in conjunction with one another. It is becoming increasingly difficult to find ghee (or clarified butter), which is butter from which water (about 20% by weight) and milk solids have been removed. It has a pleasant flavor and a very long shelf-life, lasting for years. (Ghee is also now available in a can, called "Ghee Whiz!") If you wish to make your own ghee, please follow the recipe below:

> Two-quart pot
> Stove or burner with heat control
> Silver or stainless steel spoon
> Meat thermometer
> One pound unsalted butter
> A dry one-pint container, glass or ceramic
> Two-foot square cheesecloth
> Work surface impervious to oil
> 90 minutes of unbroken time

Melt the butter in the pot, uncovered, on medium-low heat; water must evaporate.

In 3–5 minutes, the butter will melt; do not scorch. Simmer; do not let boil.

After about 20 minutes, the temperature should reach 212 °F (100 °C, boiling point of water), it should remain there for 30–40 minutes. Gently stir a few times, pushing any floating solids to the side. When all the water has gone, the temperature will rise quickly to 240 °F (116 °C). When the temperature rises, the aroma of "popcorn" appears, and the bottom of the pan will turn golden brown; TURN OFF HEAT.

While still hot strain through a cheesecloth, into a glass or ceramic pot and allow solids to drain for 2–3 minutes.

Let cool at room temperature until cool to touch. Cover and store at room temperature; do not refrigerate.

Herbal remedies: natural energy

Ayurveda prescribes a rich store of natural medicines that have been collected, tested, and recorded in medical treatises from ancient times. The tradition of collecting and preserving information about medicines in recipe books, called *Nighantus*, continued to the twentieth century (Nadkarni 1908). The most traditional source of Ayurvedic medicine is the kitchen garden. From an early stage of development, Indian medical and culinary traditions worked hand in hand with each other.

In light of the close association between food and medicine, Ayurveda classifies foods and drugs (usually vegetal) by the taste on the tongue, potency, and taste after digestion.

Rasa, taste by the tongue, is categorized into six separate tastes, with their individual elemental composition and energetic effects on the three doshas:

- *Sweet*, composed of earth and water, increases kapha and decreases pitta and vata.

- *Sour*, composed of earth and fire, increases kapha and pitta and decreases vata.

- *Saline*, composed of water and fire, increases kapha and pitta and decreases vata.

- *Pungent*, composed of wind and fire, increases pitta and vata and decreases kapha.

- *Bitter*, composed of wind and space, increases vata and decreases pitta and kapha.

- *Astringent*, composed of wind and earth, increases vata and decreases pitta and kapha.

(Zysk 1993)

Virya, potency, comprises eight types that are divided into four pairs: hot–cold, unctuous–dry, heavy–light, and dull–sharp.

Vipaka, post-digestive taste, identifies three kinds of aftertaste: sweet, sour, and pungent.

Contrary foods and drugs are always to be avoided. For instance, clarified butter and honey should not be taken in equal quantities, alkalis and salt must not be taken for a long period, milk and fish should not be consumed together, and honey should not be put in hot drinks.

Compounding

Four important criteria are considered when compounding plant substances and other ingredients into medical recipes. First, the substances that make up the recipe should have many attributes that enable it to cure several diseases, second, they should be usable in many pharmaceutical preparations, third, they should be suitable for the recipe and not cause unwanted side effects, and fourth, they should be culturally appropriate to the patients and their customs. Every medicine should be able to treat the disease's site of origin, site of manifestation, and its spread simultaneously.

A brief survey of the different kinds of medical preparations indicates the depth and content of Ayurvedic pharmaceuticals. The botanically based medicines derive largely from the Ayurvedic medical tradition, whereas the mineral and inorganic-based drugs derive from the Indian Alchemical traditions, called *Rasashastra*.

Juices are cold presses and extractions made from plants. Powders are prepared from parts of plants that have been dried in the shade and other dried ingredients. Infusions are parts of plants and herbs that have been steeped in water and strained. Cold infusions are parts of plants and herbs that were soaked in water overnight and filtered the next morning. Decoctions are vegetal products boiled in a quantity of water proportionate to the hardness of the plant part and then reduced by a fourth. It is then filtered and often used with butter, honey, or oils.

Medicated pastes and oils. Often the plant and herbal extracts are combined with other ingredients and formed into pastes, plasters, and oils. Used externally, pastes and plasters are applied for joint, muscular, and skin conditions, and oil is used for hair and head problems. Medicated oils also are used for massages and enemas.

Large and small pills and suppositories. Plant and herbal extracts are also formed into pills and suppositories to be used internally.

Alcoholic preparations are made by fermentation or distillation. Two preparations are delineated: One requires the drug to be boiled before it is fermented or distilled, and in the other, the drug is simply added to the preparation. Fifteen percent is the maximum allowable amount of alcohol content in a drug. (Zysk 1993)

Several Ayurvedic medicines are prepared from minerals and metals and are ultimately derived from ancient traditions.

Sublimates are prepared by an elaborate method leading to the sublimation of sulfur in a glass container. They are found in recipes (*Rasayanas*) used in rejuvenation therapies.

Bhasmas are ash residues produced from the calcination of metals, gems, plants, and animal products. Most are metals and minerals that are first detoxified and then purified. An important bhasma is prepared from mercury, which undergoes an 18-stage detoxification and purification process. Ayurveda maintains that bhasmas are quickly absorbed in the blood and increase the red blood cells.

Pishtis are fine powders made by trituration of gems with juices and extracts. Collyrium is made from antimony powder, lead oxide, or the soot from lamps burned with castor oil. Collyrium is used especially to improve vision. (Zysk 1993)

Of the hundreds of plants, minerals and metals mentioned in various Ayurvedic treatises, only a small selection are commonly used by the typical Ayurvedic physicians today. Similar emphasis, and some shared traditions, are illustrated in the practices of Siddha medicine in Southern India, the subject of the next chapter.

Chapter 4

Alchemical Healing

Traditional Siddha Medicine
of Southern India

Unlike Ayurveda, which has a long and detailed textual tradition in Sanskrit dating from thousands of years ago, Siddha medicine's textual history, in the Tamil language of South India, remains vague and uncertain until about the thirteenth century of the common era, when there begins evidence of medical treatises. Most of our knowledge about Siddha medicine comes from modern-day practitioners, who often maintain an unverified history of the development of their own tradition, and who, in light of the modern upsurge of Tamil pride, make fantastic claims about the age and importance of Siddha medicine vis-à-vis its closest rival in India, Ayurveda.

Based on the evidence of written secondary sources and the reports of fieldworkers in Siddha medicine, Siddha and Ayurveda share a common theoretic foundation, but differ in their respective forms of therapy. This disparity suggests that an original form of Siddha medicine may have consisted primarily of a series of treatments for specific ailments. These individual therapeutic prescriptions were later overlaid with a theoretical component from Ayurveda. In addition, diagnosis by pulse and urine, based on Ayurveda, and perhaps also Unani (see

Chapter 8), could well have been the source, in turn, for the same means of pulse and urine diagnosis.

The same pattern of medical development, which involves empirical practice followed by theory, may also apply to other forms of Indian medicine, beginning with Ayurveda itself, and including the more recent Visha Vaidya tradition of Kerala.

Siddha medicine is also distinctive in its use of *alchemy*, with fundamental principles that conform to the alchemical traditions of ancient Greece and China, and of Arabic alchemy, as reflected, for example, in Unani medicine. Siddha alchemy might well have been derived from one or a combination of these older traditions.

Ayurveda left India and found fertile ground in the West, where alternative and complementary forms of healing have become popular in recent decades. There are signs on the horizon that Siddha medicine may follow the same course. Indian systems of medicine must undergo changes and adaptations to be accommodated in a foreign environment, as in the case of Maharisha Ayurveda in the West (see Chapter 6). Some of these modifications find their way back to India, where they become integrated into the indigenous systems. Such has been the pattern of traditional medicine in most parts of the world, so that the final chapter on the history of a particular medical system can never be written. In fact, an understanding of Siddha's medical history can be revealed only in light of change and adaptation over time.

Southern sources

Looking into Siddha medicine in Tamil Nadu, Southern India, presents challenges to understanding this medical system and its history. A central problem lies with the limited availability of primary sources (akin to the "Classics" of traditional Ayurvedic or Chinese medicine) and the reliability of secondary sources prepared primarily by modern Tamil Siddha doctors. Little research on the subject has been carried out by Western students and scholars of India and Indian medicine. Even in the twenty-first century much of this mysterious medical tradition remains to be discovered.

Due to increased awareness of the Tamil language's Dravidian roots, in the second half of the twentieth century, a strong nationalist movement has grown up in Tamil Nadu. Tamils consider their cultural and linguistic heritage to be older and more important than that of the Indo-Aryans of Northern India; some even claim their ancestors comprised the first civilization on the planet. This controversy has recently been kindled by a debate centering on the still-to-be-deciphered script of the so-called Indus Valley civilization. This ancient urban culture, which extended along the Indus River and its tributaries in what is now Pakistan, resembled the great civilizations of ancient Egypt and Mesopotamia in size, development and age. One side of the debate maintains that the script represents a language probably of Dravidian origin, while the other side claims that it does not represent a language at all. Tamils, whose language is Dravidian, are anxiously following the debate, for if the former side prevails, it would confirm their antiquity on the Indian subcontinent. The lens through which Tamils look at their own history influences the image in favor of Tamil superiority and antiquity.

References to Ayurveda occur early in Tamil literature. Already in the mid-fifth century CE text, *Cilappatikara*, there is reference to Ayurveda (Tamil: *āyulvetar*). Mention of the three humors (Tamil: *tiritocam*; Sanskrit: *tridosha*) occurs in the *Tirukural*, a collection of poems that dates from around 450–550 CE.

Alchemical connections

The first Tamil Siddha text is the *Tirumandiram* written by Tirumular and dated probably to around the sixth or seventh century CE. In it there is mention of alchemy used to transform iron into gold, but no specific references to Tamil medicinal doctrines. The major sources of Siddha medicine belong to religious groups called Kayasiddhas. They seek the "perfection of the body" by means of yoga, alchemy, medicine, and certain types of Tantric religious rituals. Their works date from about the thirteenth to the fourteenth centuries CE, and are attributed to numerous authors, including *Akattiyar* (Sanskrit: *Agastya*), the traditional founder of Siddha medicine and Teraiyar (about late seventeenth century), who is said to have written twelve works on medicine. His famous disciple, Iramatevar, traveled to Mecca in the late seventeenth or early eighteenth centuries where he studied, converted to Islam, and took on the name Yakkopu (i.e., Jacob). The numerous texts on Siddha medicine which present it as a system of healing are probably not older than the sixteenth century. Therefore, Tamil Siddha medicine, as it is now exists in both theory and practice, began in Tamil Nadu around the sixteenth century, but elements of healing practices that became part of Siddha medicine, including those they hold in common with Ayurveda, came from an earlier period.

Buddhist connections

Tamil folklore surrounding healing shares a common origin with Buddhism from Northern India. Legend holds that Akattiyar performed a trephination on a sage in order to remove a toad (*terai*) from inside his skull. Akattiyar's disciple made the toad jump into a bowl of water. Because of his skill in removing the toad, Akattiyar gave the disciple the name Teraiyar, who is, however, a different person from the late seventeenth century medical author of the same name.

This legend is interesting because there is a similar account in Buddhist literature, and the legend of the toad and the cranium is a popular motif of Buddhist art and sculpture. In its earliest version found in the Pali texts of the Buddhist Canon, a skilled physician opened the cranium of a merchant from Rajagriha and removed two centipedes by touching them with a hot poker. The merchant made a full recovery. Versions of this folk story also occur in the Sanskrit literature of later Mahayana Buddhism and were translated into Tibetan and Chinese. The uniqueness of the story and its spread throughout Buddhist Asia demonstrates the influence of Buddhism in the dissemination of medical knowledge in pre-modern India.

Divine sources

Like all systems of Hindu knowledge, Siddha medicine attributes its origin to a divine source; hence its knowledge is sacred and eternal, passed down to humans for the benefit of all humanity. According to Hindu tradition, the god Shiva transmitted the knowledge of medicine to his wife Parvati, who in turn passed it on to Nandi, from whom it was given to the first practitioners of Siddha medicine. Tradition lists a total number of eighteen Siddhar practitioners, beginning with Nandi and the legendary Agattiyar through to the final Siddhar, Kudhambai. They are the acknowledged semi-mythical transmitters of Siddha medical doctrines and practices. By attributing a divine or extra-human origin to its medicine, the Tamil Siddhars have assured Siddha medicine a legitimate place in the corpus of Hindu knowledge. Although the transmission begins with Nandi, who in the form of a bull is Shiva's mode of transportation, tradition attributes the origin of medicine as well as of the Tamil language to Agattiyar.

Shiva and shakti

According to Siddha cosmology, all matter is composed of two primal forces of matter, (*shiva*) and energy (*shakti*). These two principles of existence operate in humans as well as nature, and connect the microcosm with the macrocosm. This connection is expressed by the association between the human body and the signs of the zodiac in Indian astrology, or *jyotish*. The formulation of the sequence of body parts is interesting because it follows a Babylonian and Greco-Roman system of head-to-toe correspondence (see Chapter 8 on Unani medicine) rather than an Indian one, which begins at the toes moves upwards. This formulation is illustrated in the following list, using Latin-based zodiac names (Zysk 2000).

♈ Áries (0°) = the neck

♉ Taurus (30°) = the shoulders

♊ Gémini (60°) = the arms and hands

♋ Cancer (90°) = the chest

♌ Leo (120°) = the heart and the stomach

♍ Virgo (150°) = the intestines

♎ Libra (180°) = the kidneys

♏ Scórpio (210°) = the genitals

♐ Sagittárius (240°) = the hips

♑ Capricornus (270°) = the knees

♒ Aquárius (300°) = the legs

♓ Pisces (330°) = the feet

(Zysk 2000)

In addition to this cosmic connection, which occurs in all traditions of Indian astrology (or *djoytish*), Siddha medicine relied on Ayurveda for the medical doctrines that bridge the natural world and the human body. In modern-day Siddha practice, evidence of that geneology is not always acknowledged.

There are five elements (*pañcamahabhutam*), which make up the entire natural world: solid/earth, fluid/water, radiance/fire, gas/wind, and ether/space. These elements combine in specific ways to grant the three bodily humors, called *muppini* in modern Tamil. According to Zysk (2000), they are said to be in the proportion of 1 part wind to ½ part bile to ¼ part phlegm.

- *Wind* (Tamil: *vatham*; Sanskrit: *vata*) is a combination of space and wind, and is responsible for nervous actions, movement, activity, sensations, etc. It is found in the form of the five bodily winds.

- *Bile* (Tamil: *pittam*; Sanskrit: *pitta*) is made up of fire alone and governs metabolism, digestion, assimilation, warmth, etc. Its principal seat is in the alimentary canal, from the cardiac region to small intestines. Some Ayurvedic formulations state that bile is a combination of the elements fire and water.

- *Phlegm* (Tamil: *siletuman*; Sanskrit: *shleshman, kapha*) is a combination of earth and water and is responsible for stability in the body. Its principal seats are in the chest, throat, head, and joints.

(Zysk 2000)

Next, there is the shared doctrine of the seven tissues (Tamil: *dhatu*) of the body: lymph/chyle, blood, muscle, fat, bone, marrow, and sperm and ovum. Finally, there are the five winds (Tamil: *vatham*; Sanskrit: *prana*) which circulate in the body and initiate and carry out bodily functions: *pranam* is the inhaled breath and brings about swallowing; *apanam* is the exhaled breath and is responsible for expulsion, ejection and excretion; *samanam* helps digestion; *vyanam* aids circulation of blood and nutrients; and *udanam* functions in the upper respiratory passages. There are also five secondary winds: *nagam*, the air of higher intellectual functions; *kurmam*, the air of yawning; *kirukaram*, the air of salivation; *devadhattham*, the air of laziness; and *dhananjayam*, the air that acts on death. (Zysk 2000)

Like Ayurveda, Siddha medicine maintains that the three humors predominate in humans in accordance with their nature and stage of life, and that they vary with the seasons. Every individual is born with a unique configuration of the three humors, which is called the individual's basic nature (Sanskrit: *prakriti*). It is fixed at birth and forms the basis of his or her normal, healthy state. However, during the three different stages of life and during the different seasons, one humor usually predominates. This pattern is normal, but domination by a humor must be understood in relation to the person's fundamental nature in order to maintain the balance that is the individual's basic natural state. The classification of the humors according to stages of life and seasons in Siddha differs from that found in Ayurveda. In the case of the seasons, the variation is attributed simply to the different climatic conditions that occur in the different parts of the year in the northern inland areas and the southern, Tamil coastal and inland environments.

According to Siddha, wind predominates in the first third of life, bile in the second third, and phlegm in the last third of life, while in Ayurveda phlegm dominates the first third and wind the last third of life. In terms of climate in the Indian subcontinent, the north is colder in the winter (December and January) than is the south, and the west coast has rain in June and July (with prevailing westerly winds in the northern hemisphere), when the east coast is extremely hot. A dry, cold climate is rare in the south, but it is precisely that climate which increases wind. Bile and phlegm, on the other hand, are increased when it is hot and wet.

Diagnosis: the eight features

The diagnosis of disease in Siddha medicine relies on the examination of eight anatomical features (*envagi thaervu*), which, according to Zysk (2000), are evaluated in terms of the three humors:

- *Tongue*: black indicates wind, yellow or red bile, and white phlegm; an ulcerated tongue points to anaemia.

- *Complexion*: dark indicates wind, yellow or red bile, and pale phlegm.

- *Voice*: normal indicates wind, high pitched bile, and low pitched phlegm.

- *Eyes*: muddy coloured indicates wind, yellowish or red bile, and pale phlegm.

- *Touch*: dryness indicates wind, warmness bile, and cold, clammy phlegm.

- *Stool*: black indicates wind, yellow bile, and pale phlegm.

- *Pulse*: a complex system described below.

- *Urine*: also described in detail below.

(Zysk 2000)

Pulse examination is the most emphasized diagnostic approach for modern Siddha doctors. Both diagnosis and prognosis can be obtained through this one process. These methods of diagnosis also occur in Ayurveda, but only after the fourteenth century, perhaps influenced by the introduction of Unani medicine (see

Chapter 8). Prior to this time, and in the Ayurvedic classical literature, diagnosis of disease was determined by vitiation of one or more of the humors based on observation, touch, and interrogation.

Siddha pulse diagnosis (Tamil: *natiparitchai*; Sanskrit: *nadipariksha*), like that found in Ayurveda, probably owes its origins to Unani medicine. It requires a highly developed sense of touch and refined subjective awareness. According to Siddha, the following conditions must not be present in the patient when doing a reading of the pulse:

- oily hands

- a full stomach or hunger

- physical exhaustion

- emotional distress.

If readings cannot be taken on the hand, other arterial points may be used, such as the ankle, neck, or ear lobes. It is also advisable to read the pulse at different times of the day and during different seasons of the year, since the body and mind change during the course of the day and climatic conditions affect the person's psychological and physiological states.

The pulse is felt on the female's left and male's right hand by the doctor's opposite hand, a few centimeters below the wrist joint, using the index, middle, and ring fingers. Pressure should be applied by one finger after the other beginning with the index finger. Each finger detects a particular humor, which in normal conditions has a movement representative of certain animals. The index finger feels the windy humor, which should have the movement of a swan, a cock, or a peacock; the middle finger feels the bilious humor, which should have the movement of a tortoise or a leach; and ring finger feels the phlegmatic humor, which should have the movement of a frog or a snake. Any deviation from these normal movements indicates which humor or humors are disturbed. If all humors are affected, the pulse is usually rapid with a good deal more volume than normal. After long periods of practice under the guidance of a skilled teacher, a student can begin to detect subtle differences in the flow, volume, and speed of the pulse at the point of each of the three fingers. These changes correspond to abnormalities in particular parts of the body, which the skilled Siddha doctor can pinpoint, and for which the appropriate cure can be prescribed. (Zysk 2000)

Urine examination (*muthira paritchai*) is another form of diagnosis in Siddha medicine. Not an original part of Ayurveda, urine examination probably derived from Unani medicine, where this form of diagnosis is described in early Arabic and Persian medical literature; it is also important in Tibetan medicine. Siddha practice examines the urine for its colour, smell, and texture, and further uses a technique for determining the vitiated humor by reading the distribution of a drop of gingili (sesame) oil added to the urine. The meaning of the drop's configuration is as follows: longitudinal dispersal indicates windy humor; dispersal in a ring, bilious humor; and lack of dispersal points to phlegmatic humor. A combination of two types of dispersal means that two humors are involved. Prognosis is determined by such reading as well: a slow dispersal of a drop in a circular form, or a drop that forms the shape of an umbrella, a wheel, or a jasmine or lotus blossom indicates positive prognosis. A drop that sinks, spreads rapidly with froth, splits into smaller drops and spreads rapidly, mixes with the urine, or spreads so that its pattern is that of an arrow, a sword, a spear, a pestle, a bull, or an elephant, indicates a poor prognosis.

Finally, as in Ayurveda and Unani, the condition of the eyes shows which of the humors is vitiated, as well as the patient's mental and emotional state: shifty, dry eyes point to wind; yellow eyes with photophobia indicates bile; watery, oily, eyes devoid of brightness reveals that phlegm is affected; and red, inflamed eyes show that all three humors are vitiated.

Treatment

According to traditional Siddha thinking, physicians must be knowledgeable in alchemy, astrology, and philosophy. They must be able to apply intuition and imagination. They must not seek fame or fortune from healing. They must not treat a patient before a proper diagnosis has been reached. And they must use only medicines that they have prepared themselves.

Treatment and pharmaceutics are two areas where Siddha differs considerably from Ayurveda. As in yoga (described in Chapter 5), the principal aim of Siddha medicine is to make the body perfect, not vulnerable to decay, so that the maximum term of life can be achieved. Like Ayurveda, Siddha places emphasis on positive health, so that the object of the medicine is disease-prevention and health promotion.

While traditional Ayurveda lists the following eight branches of medicine—general medicine, pediatrics, surgery, treatment of ailments above the neck, toxicology, treatment of mental disorders due to seizure by evil spirits, rejuvenation therapy, and potency therapy—Siddha medicine developed expertise in five particular branches of medicine: general medicine, pediatrics, toxicology, ophthalmology, and rejuvenation therapy. Further, while Ayurveda prescribes a therapeutic regimen involving the *Panchakarma*, purification, or "purifying actions:" emetics, purgative, enemas, bloodletting (see Chapter 3); of these Siddha employs only purgation for purification purposes.

General medicine

In Ayurveda, surgical practice forms a separate school of medicine but surgery *per se* is not a significant part of Siddha medicine. Medicated oils and pastes are applied to treat wounds and ulcers, but the use of a knife is rarely encountered at all.

Closely connected with the tradition of the martial arts in South India there developed a type of acupressure treatment based on the vital points in the human body, known as *varmam* (Sanskrit: *marman*). There are 108 points mentioned in the Ayurvedic classics, which identify them and explain that if they are injured, death can ensue. In Siddha medicine the number of important *varmam* points is also 108 (some say 107) out of a total of 400. Siddha doctors developed techniques of applying pressure to special points, called *Varmakkalai*, to remove certain ailments and of massaging the points to cure diseases. They also specialized in bone-setting and often practiced an Indian form of the martial arts, called *cilampam* or *silambattam*, which involved a kind of dueling with staffs.

According the French Institute in Pondicherry, India, the art of *varmam* is particularly widespread among the hereditary Siddha practitioners belonging to the Natar caste in the district of Kanyakumari in Tamil Nadu. The development of this special form of healing appears to have evolved naturally from the fact that the men of this caste, while carrying out their task of climbing coconut and *borassus* trees to collect the fruits and sap for toddy, occasionally fell from great heights. In order to repair the injury or save the life of a fall victim, skills of bone-setting and reviving an unconscious patient by massage developed among certain families within the caste, who have passed down their secret art from generation to generation by word of mouth. In the past, rulers employed members of this caste to cure injuries incurred in battle and to overpower their enemies by their knowledge of the Indian martial arts.

Toxicology

Toxicology as part of Siddha medicine seems to be closely linked to indigenous systems of treating snake bites and other forms of poisoning. It may have some affinity to the Visha Vaidya (poison doctor) tradition practiced by certain Nambudiri Brahmins of Kerala. Similar to this Keralan toxicological tradition, Siddha has adopted the Ayurvedic system of the three humors in order to explain the different effects of poisons; but it remains fundamentally an indigenous and local toxicological tradition. It classifies the severity and cure by means of the number of teeth or fang marks left in the victim. Four, most severe, is incurable; it implies two complete bites. One fang mark, the least severe, is cured by cold water baths and fomentation on the site of the bite. Even the bite of venomous snake may not carry venom; the more fang marks the greater likelihood that venom was injected.

Ophthalmology

Siddha medicine excels in ophthalmology. It has two separate treatises devoted to the treatment of 96 different eye diseases.

This focus may be related to the strength of Arabic optics from the Unani tradition.

Rejuvenation therapy: alchemical connection

Closely connected with Siddha yoga, the Siddha system of rejuvenation therapy, known as Kayakalpa (from Sanskrit, meaning "making the body competent for long life"), marks a distinctive feature of Siddha medicine. According to Zysk, it involves a five-step process for rejuvenating the body and prolonging life.

- Preservation of vital energy via breath control (Tamil: *vasiyogam*; Sanskrit: *pranayama*) and yoga.

- Conservation of male semen and female sexual secretions.

- Use of *muppu* or rare earth salts.

- Use of calcinated powders (Tamil: *chunnam*; Sanskrit: *bhasma*) prepared from metals and minerals.

- Use of drugs prepared from plants special to each Siddha doctor.

(Zysk 2000)

The esoteric substance called *muppu* is particular to Siddha medicine. It may be considered Siddha's equivalent of the "philosopher's stone." Its preparation is hidden in secrecy, known only by the guru, and taught only when the student is deemed qualified to accept it. It is generally thought to consist of three salts (*mu-uppu*), called *puniru*, *kallupu*, and *vediyuppu*, which correspond respectively to the sun, moon, and fire. *Puniru* is said to be a certain kind of limestone composed of globules that are found underneath a type of clay called Fuller's Earth, which contains heavy metals. In early Europe, Fuller's Earth was used by *fullers*, or those who prepared and preserved wool to weave into cloth. It is collected only on the full-moon night in April, when it is said to bubble out from the limestone. It is then purified with the use of a special herb. *Kallupu* is hard salt or stone salt, that is, rock salt, which is dug up from mines under the earth, obtained from saline deposits under the sea, or gathered from the froth of sea water that carries the undersea salt. *Kallupu* is considered to be useful in the consolidation of mercury and other metals. Finally, *vediyuppu* is potassium nitrate, which is cleaned seven times and purified with alum (aluminum salts). This magical-religious form of therapy is a common component of Siddha alchemical practice and provides a basis for the rich assortment of alchemical preparations comprising the pharmacopoeia of Siddha medicine.

Pharmacopoeia

The precise origin of the system of Siddha pharmacology is not known, but it seems to have been closely linked to the Tantric religious movement, which can be traced back to the sixth century of the common era in North India, and influenced both Buddhism and Hinduism. It was strongly anti-Brahminical, and stressed ascetic practices and religious rituals that involved "forbidden" foods and sexual practices (see Chapter 5), and often included the use of alchemical preparations.

The alchemical part of Siddha is present from at least the time of Tirumular's *Tirumandiram* (sixth or seventh century CE). Alchemy is also found in Sanskrit texts from North India, but only from about the sixth or seventh century CE. It later became an integral part of Ayurvedic medicine, called *Rasashastra*, "traditional knowledge about mercury." In the classical treatises of Ayurveda, however, mention of alchemy is absent, and only certain metals and minerals are mentioned in late classical texts from the seventh century CE. Since alchemy reached a far greater level of development in Siddha medicine than in Ayurveda, it is believed that medical alchemy may well have begun in South India among the Siddha yogins and ascetics, and was later assimilated into Ayurveda.

There are three groups of drugs in Siddha medicine: (1) inorganic substances (*thatuvargam*), (2) plant products (*mulavargam*), and (3) animal products (*jivavargam*). These drugs are all characterized by means of taste (*rasa*), quality (*guna*), potency (*virya*), post-digestive taste (*vipaka*), and specific action (*prabhava*).

Inorganic substances

Siddha has further classified the inorganic substances into six types:

- *Uppu*: twenty-five or thirty-one varieties of salts and alkalis, which are water soluble and give out vapour when heated.

- *Pashanam*: sixty-four varieties (thirty-two natural, thirty-two artificial) of non-water soluble substances that emit vapour when heated.

- *Uparasam*: seven types of non-water soluble substances that emit vapour when heated, including mica, magnetic iron, antimony, zinc sulphate, iron pyrites, ferrous sulphate and asafoetoda (*hingu*).

- *Loham*: six varieties of metals and metallic alloys that are insoluble, but melt when heated and solidify when cooled, including gold, silver, copper, iron, tin, and lead.

- *Rasam*: drugs that are soft and sublime when heated, transforming into small crystals or amorphous powders such as mercury, amalgams and compounds of mercury, and arsenic.

- *Gandhakam*: sulphur that is insoluble in water and burns off when heated.

(Zysk 2000)

Rasam and *gandhakam* combine to make *kattu*, which is a "bound" substance, that is, a substance whose ingredients are united by a process of heating.

In addition there are thirteen varieties of gems and minerals, sixteen varieties of mud and siliceous earth, thirty-five varieties of animals, and twenty-four varieties of rocks. This variety resembles the remedies of homeopathic medicine as developed in Europe during the eighteenth century.

The cornerstones of Siddha pharmacology are mercury and sulphur, which are equated to the deity Shiva and his consort Parvati, and are combined to make mercuric sulphide. Mercury, or quicksilver, is the crucial ingredient in almost every Siddha alchemical preparation. It is used in five forms (*panchasthuta*): pure mercury (*rasa*), red sulphide of mercury (*lingam*), mercuric perchloride (*viram*), mercurous chloride (*puram*), and red oxide of mercury (*rasacheduram*). Although mercury plays a key role in both the Siddha and Ayurvedic forms of medical alchemy, mercury in its pure form is not found in India and, therefore, must have become available through trade with the Roman and Byzantine empires and, subsequently, the Italian city-states of the Middle Ages. As an aside, mercury was a popular remedy in Europe until the middle of the nineteenth century, where its German name *quacksalber* gave origin to the term "quack" for those who practiced dangerous and ineffective medicine.

Siddha pharmacology combines substances that have a natural affinity to each other—such as borax and ammonia sulphate—to create a compound greater than the sum of the individual parts. This combination is called *nadabindu*, where *nada* is acidic and *bindu* is alkaline, or, in the Siddha cosmology, the female Shakti mated with the male Shiva. The most important mixture of this kind is alkaline mercury and acidic sulphur. Similarly, Siddha medicine has devised a classification of drugs as friends and foes. The former increase the curative effect, while the latter reduce it.

> Six pharmaceutical preparations are common to both Siddha and Ayurveda. They can be administered internally or on the skin. They include: calcinated metals and minerals (*chunnam*), powders (*churanam*), decoctions (*kudinir*), pastes (*karkam*), medicated clarified butter (*nei*), and medicated oils (*ennai*). Particular to Siddha medicine, however, are three special formulations: *chunnam*, metallic preparations that become alkaline, yielding calcium hydroxide, which must always be taken with another more palatable substance (*anupana*, "after drink"); *mezhugu*, waxy preparations that combine both metals and minerals; and *kattu*, inextricably bound preparations, which are impervious to water and flame. Sulphur and mercury or mercuric salts are combined to make them resistant to heat. While on the fire, certain juices are added by drops

to empower the substance. The drug can be kept for long periods and given in small doses once a day. It should not, however, be completely turned into a powder, but should be rubbed on a Sandal stone so as to yield only a few grains of the powerful substance. (Zysk 2000)

Both Ayurveda's Rasashastra, or traditional knowledge of mercury, and Siddha's alchemy have devised different methods for purifying or detoxifying metals and minerals, called *shodhana* in Sanskrit, and *suddhi murai* in Tamil, before they are reduced to ash (Sanskrit: *bhasman*; Tamil: *chunnam*). Purification is accomplished by one of two methods. One involves repeatedly heating sheets of metal and plunging them into various vegetable juices and decoctions. The other method, called "killing" (*marana*), entails destroying the metal or mineral by the use of powerful herbs, so that it loses its identity and becomes converted into fine powders with the natures of oxides or sulphides, which can be processed by the intestinal juices. After this purification procedure, the metal or mineral is combined with its appropriate acid or alkaline, and is prepared for its final transformation into an ash or "bhasman" by incineration in special furnaces made of cow-dung cakes (replaced by electric ovens in modern establishments!).

According to Zysk, there are nine principles that must be followed in the calcination of metals and minerals:

1. There is no alchemical process without mercury.

2. There is no fixation without alkali.

3. There is no colouring without sulphur.

4. There is no quintessence without copper sulphate.

5. There is no animation without conflagration.

6. There is no calcination without corrosive lime.

7. There is no compound without correct blowing.

8. There is no fusion without suitable flux.

9. There is no strong fluid without salammoniac.

(Zysk 2000)

The traditional incineration process may vary slightly among different Siddha doctors, but all procedures require repeated heating in a fire fueled by dung patties. The number of burnings can reach one hundred for certain preparations. In traditional Ayurveda, the duration and intensity of the heat is regulated by the size of the pile of dung, called a *puta* in Sanskrit. Siddha medicine devised a method with a special substance made of inorganic salts, in Tamil called *jayani*, which reduces the number of burnings to only three or four. In order to increase the potency of the ash (*chunnam*), Siddha practitioners add the esoteric substance *muppu*, which seems to vary in individual composition from one Siddha doctor to another. Other ingredients added to increase a *chunnam*'s potency are healthy human urine (*amuri*), or urine salts (*amuriuppu*) obtained from the evaporation of large quantities of urine. Neither of these additives is found in Ayurveda's Rasashastra.

According to Zysk, in modern Siddha medicine different metals have different healing effects:

- *Mercury* is antibacterial and antisyphilitic (and was used for this purpose in the West until the early twentieth century).

- *Sulphur* is used against scabies and skin diseases, rheumatoid arthritis, spasmodic asthma, jaundice, blood poisoning, and internally as a stool softener.

- *Gold* is effective against rheumatoid arthritis, and as a nervine tonic, an antidote, and a sexual stimulant.

- *Arsenic* cures all fevers, asthma, and anaemia.

- *Copper* is used to treat leprosy, skin diseases, and to improve the blood.

- *Iron* is effective against anaemia, jaundice, and as a general tonic for toning the body.

(Zysk 2000)

This kind of knowledge about the healing properties of various minerals was ultimately carried into the use of mineral baths, spas and water therapies in the West.

Despite the scientific evidence that shows many of these inorganic substances—minerals and metals—to be toxic to the human body, both Siddha and Ayurvedic practitioners continue to use them in their everyday treatment of patients. They claim that their respective traditions have provided special techniques to detoxify the metals and minerals and to render them safe and extremely potent. Again, as in the practice of homeopathy, certain biologically active substances that are toxic in one form or dose may be prepared so that its beneficial effects predominated.

Plant products

In terms of herbal drugs, Siddha practitioners drew upon a *materia medica* of over a hundred plants and plant products, some of which are imported from as far away as the Himalaya (see Chapter 7). These herbal remedies are used for three purposes in Siddha medicine. First, as mentioned earlier, certain drugs purify the minerals and metals before they are transformed into ash. Second, many plants and plant substances are used to eliminate waste products from the body through a process of body purification involving purgation of the nose and throat, enemas and laxatives, and the removal of toxins from the skin by the application of medicated pastes. This procedure resembles the process of the five methods of purification (Sanskrit: *pañcakarman*) in Ayurveda. Third, plants are used to treat specific ailments, and for the general toning or tonification of the body.

Animal products

Siddha doctors also used animal products, such as human and canine skulls and bones, in the preparation of a special "ash" or *chunnam* (Tamil: *peranda chunnam*), which is said to be effective against mental disorders. The preparation of bone ash would serve to alkalinize (make basic versus acidic) any mixtures and unbind various active principles that might otherwise not be metabolically available. A clear example from American Indian ethnomedicine is the use of ash, or mineral lime from seashells, to alkanize (make basic versus acidic) maize, allowing the B vitamins such as niacin to become unbound and available for metabolism when ingested.

Ayurvedic pharmaceutical manufacturers in India have begun to adopt the Western system of "good manufacturing procedures," and to resort to Ayurveda's rich pharmacopoeia of plant-based medicines, in order to make their products more accessible to a Western clientele. Such is not the case with Siddha medicine, which has yet to experience the financial rewards that come from serving Western markets.

Both Siddha and Ayurveda are sophisticated systems of medicine, practiced in India for more than 2500 years. Traditional medicine in India focuses on the whole organism and its relation to the external world to reestablish and maintain the harmonious balance that exists within the body and between the body and its environment. Few reliable sources for traditional Ayurveda have been available in English. Most of the accurate works are by and for specialists, and are virtually inaccessible to the reader without knowledge of Sanskrit (e.g., Meulenbeld 1974; Srikanta Murthy 1984). This circumstance suggests that many of the mysteries of Ayurvedic and Siddha healing are yet to be uncovered, and may hold yet greater promise than has yet been realized.

Chapter 5

Yoga

A Journey from Body to Spirit

Yoga is a textual and practical tradition that developed in ancient India. Its origins can be traced in classic writings, as well as in traditions passed down over time. It is important to understand that in the traditional Indian context, yoga is an expression of a philosophical system, the same system, with the same central idea of vital energy as in Ayurveda. In Ayurveda, the focus of expression is physical health, while in yoga, the focus is body-mind development leading to the full realization of the spirit.

A wide range of modalities and techniques of yoga have developed to facilitate this journey on life's path. These techniques, which reflect the many facets of the human experience of body, mind, and spirit, include postural stretching and exercise, moral action in the world, devotional practice, meditation, and sexual practices. Yoga can be utilized as complementary medicine, but as with the practice of Ayurveda, it encompasses a broader philosophical system and lifestyle, in addition to those modalities that may represent specific therapies.

Traditional Ayurveda may have developed separately from the tradition of yoga in India, each coming down through the centuries with perceivable influences of one upon the other. On the other hand, it may be seen that yoga practice has incorporated aspects of Ayurvedic medicine to help maintain the healthy bodily condition necessary for spiritual development.

In the current environment, there may be special teacher–student relationships in which the yogi (one who knows yoga) acts as the mentor (or, literally, the *guru*) to impart knowledge of yoga philosophy and technique to the pupil. Formulary versions of hatha yoga, for example, in which the physical postures and techniques are taught without the philosophical foundation, would not properly be considered yoga, but rather physical training and physical therapy, which nonetheless may be beneficial.

The yoke is on you

Yoga is a common word in Sanskrit, one of the most ancient Indo-European languages. It has a range of meanings: conjunction, constellation, team, or union. The term is related to words in other Indo-European languages, including the Latin *iugum*, German *joch*, and English *yoke*, all of which share meaning. According to the Advaita Vedanta, yoga is characteristic of philosophical teachings that subscribe to a non-dualist metaphysical reality in which the individual self (*atman*) is seen as ultimately identical with the transcendental self (*paramatman*) underlying all phenomena. However, there is also a dualist school, known as raja yoga, or classical yoga, founded by the semi-mythical Patanjali. In this case, yoga focuses not so much on the union with ultimate reality but on disunion or separation from the ego. The ultimate outcome is similar, because when the yoga practitioner succeeds in transcending the ego, he or she simultaneously realizes the true essence of the self or soul. Thus, yoga comprises schools that embrace total renunciation of the world (*samnyasa*), those that encourage proper performance of one's duty in the world (*karma*), schools that regard dispassionate wisdom (*dhyana*) as the means to spiritual enlightenment, and those that place love and devotion above all else (*bhakti*). One may observe these same ranges of expression within other spiritual traditions, such as Judaism, Islam, and very clearly by considering the uniquely varied spiritual expressions in the religious orders of Roman Catholicism. Although different versions of yoga are more or less religious and ritualistic, all are spiritual, and yoga may be regarded, perhaps, as India's common brand of spirituality.

Ancient knowledge: the Vedas, epics, and Upanishads

Evidence of yoga beliefs and practices may be observed in the ancient Rigveda (or knowledge of praise), which serves as a source of the sacred heritage of Hinduism. It is the oldest of the four Vedas (veda means knowledge), dating back to about 1200 BCE, the others being the Samaveda, the Yajurveda, and the Atharvaveda. The Vedas comprise classic Sanskrit texts said to have been heard (*shruta*) by, and thereby revealed to, seers (*rishi*). The texts take the form of poems or hymns based on the mystical visions, ecstasies, and insights of the Rishis, and are traditionally regarded as "revealed wisdom." Yogins within the Hindu tradition based their practice and teaching on this Vedic revelation. Others, such as Gautama the Buddha and Mahavira, the founders of Buddhism and Jainism, respectively, began within the tradition, and then were seen to have deviated from the revealed wisdom of the texts. In essence, the Buddha's "noble eightfold path" presents an early form of non-Vedic yoga.

The *Bhagavad Gita* (Lord's Song), the best known and treasured of all yoga scriptures, dates to approximately 500 BCE. Mahatma Gandhi referred to it as "my mother." It is embedded in the *Mahabharata*, one of the two major Hindu epics (the other being the *Ramayana*). It tells the story of a great war between two ancient Indian peoples, the Kurus and the Pandavas. Its mythical author, Vyasa, weaves spiritual teachings into the account of the events leading up to the war, the eighteen-day war itself, and its aftermath. The tale of the *Bhagavad Gita* begins on the morning of the first battle, when the Pandava prince, Arjuna, refuses to fight because he finds teachers and friends among the ranks of the enemy. Krishna, appearing in a divine incarnation as Arjuna's charioteer, encourages to him to do his duty because this is a "just war" to restore moral order. Yoga teachings are also given elsewhere in the *Mahabharata.*

During the period 500 BCE to about 100 CE, many Upanishads containing yoga teachings were composed. The Upanishads are esoteric and philosophical scriptures describing the way to self-understanding, transcendence, and union with the universe. Wisdom is seen as the supreme means to this goal. Wisdom is distinct from knowledge, which relies empirically on the senses, and grasps knowledge from the outside. The spiritual discipline of wisdom is represented in dhyana yoga. "Classical" yoga emerged in about 200 CE, as codified by Patanjali in the famous Yoga Sutras, or aphorisms of yoga.

Later (post-classical) sources of yogic knowledge are the Tantras (or webs), which belong to the tradition of Shiva-Shakti worship. Shiva manifests the universal male principle and is usually worshiped as a Hindu god; Shakti, meaning "power," refers to female principle or energy in the world, usually visualized as a goddess. Tantric yoga is concerned with enlisting this goddess energy in the yogic process. Yoga is also an integral part of Shiva worship, as given in the Agamas (traditions).

Hatha yoga (or forceful yoga) is an important tradition that emerged in the eleventh century, under the influence of Tantra, and has its own scriptures, including the Geranda-Samhita and the Shiva-Samhita.

Swami Vivekananda was a nineteenth-century yogin in the Hindu tradition of Advaita Vedanta, a non-dual system of thought and practice drawn from the Vedic texts. He spoke well to the West; in fact, he represented Hinduism at the World Parliament of Religions in 1894. The understanding he promoted foreshadows insights of contemporary Western science:

> Every particle in the body is continually changing; no one has the same body for many minutes together, and yet we think of it as the same body. So with the mind: one moment it is happy, another moment unhappy; one moment strong, another weak—an ever changing whirlpool. That cannot be the Spirit which is infinite... Any particle in this universe can change in relation to any other particle. But take the universe as one; then in relation to what can IT

move? There is nothing besides IT. So this infinite unit is unchangeable, immovable, absolute, and this is the Real Man [sic].

The Real Man (or Woman) of Vivekananda is the eternal gender-transcending subject, the essential self of all beings and things. The insights of twentieth-century fundamental physics, as well as much of the knowledge of human physiology, biology, and pathology (see Chapters 1 and 2), came in large measure after Swami Vivekananda's talks of 1894.

Human suffering and spirit

Since the beginning, practitioners of yoga have cultivated the ideal of "renunciation" (*samnyasa*). Some interpret this practice to imply abandoning worldly life altogether. Others take renunciation primarily as an inner attitude. To the practitioner of dhyana yoga, renunciation comes naturally as a realization of the true pattern of life and nature of reality.

Yogic philosophy holds that human suffering is caused by *kleshas*, or afflictions, which are:

1. ignorance, or unawareness of reality

2. ego

3. attraction towards objects

4. repulsion from objects

5. fear of death.

At the same time, yoga realizes that these kleshas are not independent, but that one leads to the next—the root cause being ignorance. Being unaware of the ultimate reality of connectedness gives rise to a sense of a separate identity or ego. Things and people that strengthen the ego sense are found attractive, so the ego clings to them and fears their loss, which brings suffering, Things and people that weaken the ego sense are considered repulsive, so the ego pushes them away and fears their appearance, which also brings suffering. The identification with the ego sense inherently brings with it a deep aversion to death and the consequent loss of ego identity.

Reduction of the kleshas is an aim of yoga, as a predominance of kleshas is detrimental to progress on the spiritual path. As one progresses and evolves along the spiritual path, one realizes that one's view of life in the present state of consciousness is far inferior to the more subtle essence, which slowly reveals itself.

Karma

Ancient Vedic spirituality was based on the ideal of outward sacrifice combined with inward meditation. The later Upanishads prescribed meditation as an inner sacrifice. This distinction was traditionally couched in terms of wisdom (dhyana) versus action (karma). To the dhyana yogin, the greater wisdom may be in non-action. The growth of the attractiveness of non-action as a path began to concern social leaders in India by the middle of the first millennium CE. They then argued that a person should wait until his or her social duties to household and family were fulfilled before retiring to the mountain top (an early and literal form of retirement). Indian lawgivers favored a lifestyle unfolding in four phases (ashrama): (1) student, (2) householder, (3) forest-dweller (in late maturity), and (4) freely wandering ascetic (in old age).

The follower of karma yoga acts in daily life so as to lessen lawlessness and restore virtue (dharma) or harmony. Like Mahatma Gandhi, the karma yogin works for the welfare of others. Devotionally, this practice may focus on the worship of God in personal form, notably Lord Krishna.

Although love and devotion are central to Krishna's message, it is unthinkable without the corollaries of action and wisdom. As a divine incarnation, Krishna is born whenever the moral order has collapsed and the world is enveloped in spiritual darkness. Krishna's karma yoga is sometimes used to justify military action. It must be remembered that the war Krishna encouraged Arjuna to fight against the Kurus had the specific purpose of restoring moral order. The karma yogin may be seen as a "warrior" in this sense, whose good fight is manifest in the material world.

The link between karma yoga and meditation is the loss of identification with the ego while performing one's karma as the instrument of the supreme consciousness. When the individual no longer considers the ego to be the actor, but merely the instrument, the work becomes spiritualized. Desires and mental problems automatically disappear, as do likes and dislikes, which otherwise create obstacles to meditation. Also, karma yoga further develops the faculty of concentration and the will. Briefly, the will can be defined as the ability to harmonize, motivate, and mobilize all one's abilities and actions to achieve a definite aim.

Bhakti: devotion

Bhakti means "devotion," generally devotion to God or the supreme consciousness in one of its manifestations. These manifestations may be one of numerous avatars or divine incarnations, or may also be one's guru or anyone or anything that evokes strong emotions of reverence. Instead of directing the attention to an impersonal form of consciousness, as in raja yoga and dhyana yoga, one's love is directed to something more tangible and concrete.

It is generally accepted that individuals are continually trying to find someone or something to which they can totally direct their emotion and devotion, and that this search carries on continually through life. In bhakti yoga the state of meditation arises because the person who feels devotion automatically concentrates her or his mind, depending on the degree of devotion. This also results in the person losing awareness of "I-ness" or ego. Ideally, bhakti yoga alone can be sufficient to bring about higher states of meditation, and no other practice is necessary. Important components of bhakti yoga include the following:

- *Sravana*, or hearing of the glories of God.
- *Nama sankirtan*, or repetition of God's name(s).
- *Smarana*, or remembrance of God.
- *Vandana*, or prayers to God.
- *Archana*, or ritualistic worship of God.

Although a devotional attitude in spiritual life is reflected in the writings of the seers of the Vedas, an independent path of bhakti yoga emerged in the middle of the first millennium and centered on the theistic religions worshiping Krishna (a divine incarnation of Vishnu) and Shiva. Bhakti yoga draws from verses of the *Bhagavad Gita*. Shiva worshipers in the same era created the Shvetashvatara Upanishad as a devotional text. The bhakti yogin devotes himself or herself to the constant remembrance of the divine in all things. As mentioned, this worship takes the form of rituals, love-intoxicated chanting, singing, dancing, and meditation.

Raja yoga

Also known as classical yoga, raja yoga was formulated by Patanjali in the Yoga Sutra around 200 BCE. This school is considered one of the six orthodox systems of Hindu philosophy; raja yoga provides the most systematic access to the full range of practical dimensions of yoga. Patanjali enumerated eight principal limbs of practice as follows:

1. moral restraint: gentleness, truthfulness, honesty, chastity, and generosity (the *yamas*, or social code)

2. discipline: purity, contentment, asceticism, study, and devotion (the *niyamas*, or observances)

3. posture (*asana*)

4. breathing (*pranayama*)

5. withdrawal of the senses (*pratyahara*)

6. concentration (*dharana*)

7. meditation (*dhyana*)

8. ecstasy (*samadhi*).

These eight limbs are seen as stages for progressive steps toward attainment of successful meditation and indicate how obstacles on the spiritual path can be overcome.

The social and personal codes of conduct (yamas and niyamas) prepare the mind and body for the higher stages of meditation, by reducing attachment and inducing tranquility.

Asanas, or yogic postures, provide steady and comfortable positions for the body to facilitate and practice concentration and meditation without physical disturbance. Any position of the body that is even slightly uncomfortable will result in preoccupation of the mind with the body. At the same time, other asanas are more therapeutic than meditational. These therapeutic asanas are helpful in treatment and prevention of certain diseases of both body and mind. They also help induce tranquillity of mind, thereby encouraging successful meditation practice.

The word *prana* is often used in yoga, and is often misunderstood to mean only "breath." Prana denotes "life force" or vital energy (see Chapter 2). Yoga also sees it as the medium through which matter and mind are linked to consciousness. The aim of the breathing techniques of pranayama is control over the flow of prana, which is intimately linked to the breathing process. Pranayama results in redistribution of prana in the body, enabling the mind to ascend to the next stages of concentration.

Pratyahara is a method to withdraw the mind from association with the external world so that it can go to the stage of dharana and dhyana. This detachment is accomplished by reducing to zero the selection of sense impressions that are communicated to the mind. The mind is often likened to a naughty child, who does the opposite of what one wants the child to do. This idiosyncracy of the mind is used for pratyahara, in which the mind is forced to think of external things with the eyes closed; in time, the mind tends to lose interest in the external sounds and does not associate with sense impressions—"out of sight, out of mind." Antarmouna is a pratyahara technique that specifically exploits this behavior of the mind. Pratyahara also requires that the sitting posture, or asana, be comfortable. Many techniques involve a systematic rotation of the awareness around different parts of the body, or awareness of the breathing process, or awareness of sounds uttered either mentally or verbally. This satisfies the wandering tendency of the mind in a controlled manner.

Dharana, or concentration, is the method to eliminate memories of the past and projections of future events by concentrating totally on one object to the exclusion of all others. In yogic concentration the mind is not held completely rigid; the processes of the mind are not curtailed. The mind is held so that it is aware of one object, but it should move in the sense that it realizes deeper aspects of the object not perceivable earlier.

Dhayana is an extension of dharana and has been defined by Patanjali as the uninterrupted flow of concentration of mind on the object of meditation or concentration. The difference between dharana and dhyana is that in dharana the practitioner has to bring back the awareness to the object of concentration, while in dhyana the mind has been subjugated and is totally and continually absorbed in the object. Samadhi is the fullest extension of dhyana and is the climax of meditation. Patanjali has defined samadhi as that state in which there is only consciousness of the object and no concurrent consciousness of the mind.

The stages from dharana to samadhi are actually different names for different degrees of attainment. One automatically and spontaneously leads to the next; these are not totally different practices as are the lower five stages. However, it is at these stages that the master or "guru" becomes a necessity for guiding the aspirant safely. Safety is also a concern in practicing and accessing the potency of the next form of yoga, kundalini.

Kundalini

In accordance with ancient writings, kundalini yoga was designed to awaken the "serpent power" or spirit within the body. At present, kundalini awakenings may be classified under the medical category of "spiritual emergence," which is considered a psychological crisis. In *The Kundalini Experience* (1976), American psychiatrist Lee Sannella argued that such "awakenings" should be considered spiritual rather than psychiatric in nature.

The Sanskrit word kundalini is the feminine form of kundala, meaning "ring" or "coil." It thus means "she who is coiled," like a serpent. This is an appropriate metaphor for its psychospiritual potential. Its power is conceived as the goddess counterpart of Shiva, which is pure consciousness.

Each level of the mind is associated with a psychic center, or chakra (see below). The aim of kundalini yoga is to overcome usual inactivity of the higher chakras so that they are stimulated and the individual is able to experience higher levels of the mind. The basic method of awakening these psychic centers in kundalini yoga is deep concentration on the centers and willing their arousal.

A fully awakened kundalini is said actually to restructure the body, leading to a reordering of control over vital functions, such as pulse, intestinal contractions, and brain activity. In hatha yoga (see below), various techniques are used to accomplish these results by focusing the life breath or life force (prana) through mental concentration and controlled breathing. Because kundalini is thought to be dormant in the lowest chakra of the energetic body, effort is concentrated on that particular spot.

Chakras

The energetic body in yoga is thought to consist of between five and seven energy centers, or chakras (literally, "wheels"). In hatha yoga and many Tantric schools of yoga, the seven energy centers are, in ascending order, as follows:

1. *Muladhara*: "root-prop wheel," situated in the perineum (yoni), corresponding to the sacrococcygeal nerve plexus, associated with the earth element—the resting place of dormant kundalini.

2. *Svadhishthana*: "own-base wheel," located in the genitals, corresponding to the sacral plexus at the fourth lumbar vertebra, associated with the water element.

3. *Manipura*: "jewel-city wheel," located at the navel, corresponding to the solar plexus, associated with fire.

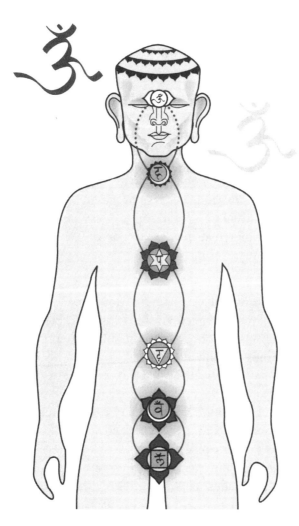

Figure 5.1 Yogic psychic anatomy

4. *Anahata*: "wheel of the unstruck," located at the heart, corresponding to the cardiac plexus, associated with the air element.

5. *Vishuddhi*: "wheel of purity," located at the throat, corresponding to the laryngeal plexus, associated with the ether element.

6. *Ajna*: "command wheel," located in the brain, corresponding to the vestigial third eye (known as the eye of Shiva, or the pineal gland in Western medicine), associated with the mind.

7. *Sahasrara*: "thousand-spoked wheel," located at the crown, associated with non-local consciousness.

These chakras as conceptualized here may be seen as illustrating two fundamental insights of yoga: matter is a low velocity form of vibrational energy that exists in states of high velocity elsewhere, and consciousness is not inevitably bound in matter but is inherently free (see Chapter 1). Kundalini yoga is a method for finding that freedom of consciousness.

Nadis

The word *nadi* means a "current" or "flow," connecting the different chakras and other psychic centers. There are said to be 72,000 such nadis; those of particular importance are the sushumna, pingala, and ida nadis.

Sushumna is by far the most important nadi. With its base at the mooladhara chakra, it travels through the spinal column and terminates at the center of the Sahasrara chakra via the swadhishthana, manipura, anahata, and vishuddhi chakras. It is in this nadi that the kundalini flows when it is awakened.

The pingala and ida nadis start at the muladhara and terminate at the ajna chakra, crossing the sushumna at the swadhishthana, manipura, anahata, and vishuddhi chakras in a serpent-like fashion, forming semicircular curves between two consecutive chakras. The pingala or "solar" nadi starts with a right curve from the muladhara; the ida or "lunar" nadi starts with a left curve from the muladhara.

Hatha yoga

Hatha means "force" or "forceful," and refers to the practice of yoga that uses physical purification and body strengthening as an arduous means of self-transformation and transcendence. A frail or diseased body may prove an obstacle on the path to enlightenment of the spirit and therefore must be properly trained.

Physical and mental training and fitness are important because at the core of hatha yoga is the potentially dangerous process of awakening the kundalini Shakti. This arousal of the power of consciousness at the lowest chakra and transmission to the highest chakra is tremendously powerful—physically and mentally.

Historically, hatha yoga is based on the development of tantra yoga (described below). Long before the emergence of hatha yoga, the awakening of kundalini Shakti was central to tantric esotericism. In fact, one school of thought holds that in the word *hatha*, *ha* stands for the ida nadi and *tha* stands for the pingala nadi. It is held that when the flow of prana in ida is equal to the flow of prana in pingala, kundalini automatically starts to rise. Therefore, hatha yoga is concerned with the two nadis, ida and pingala, and its aim is balancing the flow of prana in each nadi. When the kundalini is activated in this way, it stimulates the chakras, and meditation and spiritual realization automatically take place.

Many of the hatha yoga practices also attempt to directly stimulate the chakras and to clean and generally improve the condition of various physical organs that are linked to the chakras. In preparation, hatha yoga incorporates many techniques for cleansing and stabilization of body energy. It includes many postures or positions (*asanas*) to maintain or restore well-being, to improve vitality and flexibility, and to facilitate prolonged meditation. The basis is breathing and breath control (*pranayama*), and various techniques are used to modulate the body's vital winds (*prana*) through the breath. This form of yoga is the best known in the West, although its deeper philosophical foundations are rarely understood or practiced. It is widely reduced in its conceptualization to another form of "fitness training," although its effects are more far reaching.

The twentieth-century hatha yoga master B.K.S. Iyengar, who trained many American hatha yoga teachers, said, "The original idea of yoga is freedom and beatitude, and the by-products...including physical health, are secondary for the practitioner."

Hatha yoga entails a complex program of physical cleansing (shodhana). The Geranda-Samhita describes six acts, as follows:

1. *Dhauti* (cleansing), consisting of four techniques: inner, dental, "heart" or chest, and "base" purification. "Inner cleansing" uses four exercises: swallowing the breath and expelling it through the anus, filling the stomach with water, stimulating the abdominal "fire" by repetitions of contracting the navel against the spine, and washing the prolapsed intestines (not medically recommended). "Dental cleansing" covers the teeth, tongue, ears, and frontal sinuses. "Heart cleansing" consists of induced or self-induced emesis. "Base cleansing" is manual cleansing of the anus with water or other solution.

2. *Vasti or basti*: bladder cleansing by contracting the urinary sphincter, usually while standing in water.

3. *Neti*: threading a thin cloth through the nostril and out the mouth to remove mucus and "open up the third eye."

4. *Lauli or nauli*: rolling the abdominal muscles sideways to massage the inner organs.

5. *Trataka*: gazing steadily at a small, close object, such as a candle flame, until tears flow, to develop the powers of concentration.

6. *Kapala-bhati*: three practices involving breathing in through the right nostril and out through the left (and vice versa), drawing water through the nostrils and expelling it through the mouth, and sucking water up through the mouth and expelling it through the nose. This is done to purify the frontal portion of the brain.

Relaxation, as with purification, is another important preparatory aspect involving the postures (asanas) of hatha yoga. Relaxation applies not only to the body but also to the mind. When posture is cultivated properly, it creates the sensation that the body is loosening up and widening out. Thus, posture is more than gymnastics or acrobatics; it is the art of relaxation to the point of meditation and beyond. Following are some postures for meditation:

- *Siddha-asana*, the "successful posture," is achieved by pressing the left heel against the perineum and placing the right foot above the genitals.

  ○ *Padmasana*, the "lotus posture," is achieved by placing the right foot on the left thigh and the left foot on the right thigh. The classic texts also teach crossing the arms behind the back and grasping the left toe with the left hand and the right toe with the right hand, called the bound lotus. The lotus posture, in addition to promoting relaxation, is said to alleviate a number of diseases. It often is seen in depictions of the Buddha.

- *Sukhasana*, the "happy posture," favored by many Americans, is widely known as the tailor's seat.

Other well-known postures are the tree, triangle, hands-to-feet, adamantine, cow-face, back-stretching, serpent (cobra), all-limb, plow, and head postures.

In addition to the postures, hatha yoga has a series of bandhas (bonds or locks) and mudras (seals). There are three principal types of locks, in which the life force is forcibly retained in the body. The root lock is the contraction of the anal sphincter. The upward lock is executed by pulling the stomach up until there is a hollow below the rib cage, said to force the vital energy upward "like a great bird." The throat contraction lock is done by placing the chin down against the collarbone, stopping the downward flow of "ambrosial fluid" (possibly a reference to hormonal secretions). It prevents the life force (and the vital breath) from escaping through the nose or mouth.

The hatha yoga seals consist of eight important techniques:

1. *Space-seal*: turning the tongue back and inserting it in the nasopharynx (cavity at the back of the mouth leading to the nose), possible only if the frenulum underneath the tongue has been deliberately cut. This mudra is said to satisfy hunger, quench thirst, cure disease, and postpone death.

2. *Power-stirring*: contracting the anus and forcing the vital energy into the central channel at the lowest chakra, the seat of the kundalini.

3. *Shambu*: a meditation technique more than a physical exercise, it requires a wide-eyed, unfocused gaze. Shambu, another name for Shiva, is regarded as the revealer of the secrets of Tantrism.

4. *Vajroli*: sucking released semen back into the urethra. Females also learn this technique so as not to waste the valuable hormonal and chemical properties of semen.

5. *Sahajoli*: rubbing ejaculated semen into the skin.

6. *Amaroli*: drinking the midflow of the urine, thought to have certain healing properties.

7. *Womb*: while seated in the siddha-asana posture, with eyes, ears, and nostrils closed with the ten fingers, the body's energy is forced through the six chakras by means of breath control, mantra, and visualization.

8. *Six openings*: placing the thumbs on the two ears, the index and middle fingers on the two eyes, and the ring and the little fingers on the two nostrils.

Similarly, there are eight major breathing techniques (*pranayama*) for modulating the flow of vital energy into the body. Incorrect pranayama may cause hiccups, asthma, headache, and other ailments.

Meditation

Although Western adoptions and adaptations of yoga practices have placed great emphasis on body postures, with little attention to meditation, such forms of inner cultivation actually are central to the achievement of the common goal of the myriad of yoga paths—spiritual realization. Meditation is described and recommended in the early texts, where the terms that came to be most associated with the practices are *dhyana* and *bhavana*. Dhyana, meaning meditation or thought, is the term that when transliterated gave the names to many of the forms of Buddhist meditation—the Buddha yoga—established across Asia, from *Chan* in China, to *Son* in Korea, *Zen* in Japan, and *Thien* in Vietnam. Bhavana, meaning cultivation, is a term that suggests the ongoing, incremental work of meditation, as well as its potential flowering.

The centrality of meditation to yoga can be seen easily in its position in Patanjali's eight-limbed classical yoga formulation, delineated above under raja yoga. Dhyana is the penultimate limb. It deepens the concentration of *dharana*, which comes before, and creates the conditions for the ecstasy and absorption of *samadhi*, which is the final limb. Indeed, all of the limbs contribute to the journey to spiritual realization.

Meditation, inherently, is a practice of mind and body. Sitting postures (*asana* is Sanskrit for "seat") are favored and perhaps are emblematic of the body in meditation in the popular Western imagination; however, the meditator may assume any posture. The activity of the mind is concentrated on an object. Here again, certain objects, such as the ongoing breath or a chosen word or sound (*mantra*), define the popular view, yet the choice of objects is without limit. Depending upon his or her tradition and intention, the meditator may focus on, for example, the body and its parts and processes, the workings of the mind and emotions, the vital energy and its channels and organs, the kundalini force, the teacher (*guru*), images and qualities of blissful or even wrathful deities, abstract concepts, or the transcendental self. As concentration deepens through practice, the meditator experiences physical benefits, the slow, efficient breathing and heart rate; lowered muscle tension and blood pressure; and other benefits of the para-sympathetic response. (The Harvard cardiologist Herbert Benson brought this aspect of meditation to prominence in evidence-based Western medicine in his adaptation of mantra-focused meditation as *The Relaxation Response*, the title of his 1976 book.) Deepening further, the meditator may experience a sense of peace that overflows into everyday life, and the possibility for absorptive or non-dual experience that begins the process of spiritual realization.

Meditation is an ongoing process. It is considered important to have a secure environment for meditation, where interruptions can be minimized. Having an established location reserved for meditation and yoga is helpful, as repeated meditation in the same place may help develop an energetic imprint that facilitates the meditative state.

Time of day is important. As with location, it is useful to meditate at a consistent time each day, regardless of which particular moment is chosen. Most traditions indicate that early morning is the best time to meditate. Yogins in India typically meditate at sunrise, known as the hour of Brahma. Other recommended times include noon, sunset, and midnight.

It is advised, at the outset, to sit in meditation for no more than 15 minutes at a time, and to increase the duration as concentration is cultivated. Initially the desire for sleep or mental indulgence in fantasies or daydreaming may tend to replace the meditative state. With this sense that a level of effort is required, being well rested is important for meditation, as it is for general health, because tiredness invites sleep or daydreaming. Sexual activity should be avoided shortly before meditation because it may deplete the vital energy in the psychoenergetic centers (*chakras*).

Mantras

The consciousness-altering effects of sound are well known and probably belong to the earliest expression of human culture. Sacred sounds preceded yoga and were most likely part of the early Vedic rituals and religion.

Some of the mystical insights and writings of the ancient Vedic sages have been reinterpreted in light of modern understanding of fundamental physics, for example, that the universe is "an ocean of vibrations." According to the schools of Siddha yoga, also known as mantra yoga, all perceptible sounds ultimately derive from a universal matrix of sound. This expression has been translated as "sonic absolute," which is typically articulated as the monosyllabic sound "OM (or AUM)." Classic physics states that sounds are waves of consecutive compressions and rarefactions of air or other fluid.

Mantra yoga uses the vehicle of sonic vibration to unify consciousness through recitation and contemplation of special numinous sounds such as OM. In addition, the monosyllables HAM, YAM, RAM, VAM, LAM, AH, HUM, and PHAT are also used.

Few mantras have a denotative meaning, but, rather, are used to produce specific states of energy and consciousness. After continuous and dedicated practice, the mantra is repeated automatically without strain or effort. The mantra spontaneously manifests itself and becomes an integral part of the mind. The mind vibrates with the sound of the mantra. This approach provides a powerful means of attaining meditational states, since the mind is rendered calm and concentrated. The mantra acts as a pathway between normal states of consciousness and superconsciousness.

Mental imagery

Similar to many mind-body interventions, yoga employs visualization as one of the traditional forms of meditation. Visualization has been practiced particularly in the Tantric Buddhism of Tibet (see Chapter 7). Deity yoga involves the visualization of deities and is the essential practice of what is called highest toga tantra. Deities are usually visualized together with their respective environments, known as *mandalas*, or "circles."

Tantra

Tantric yoga posits that sexual energy is an important reservoir that should be used wisely to facilitate the spiritual process rather than block it through orgasmic release.

There are right-handed and left-handed practices of Tantric yoga. In left-handed Tantra, sexual union is a central ritual. In many countries throughout the Middle East (see Chapter 8 on Unani medicine) and South Asia, the left hand is the taboo hand used for private bodily functions, not for eating or greeting. (The Latin term *sinister* also means "left.") In left-handed Tantra, things that are taboo are charged with energy because of the constant, negative attention they receive. This yoga makes a point of breaking with established norms by using taboo functions such as sexuality in the service of spiritual transformation.

At the center of left-handed Tantra are the five prohibitions: sex, wine, meat, fish, and parched grain. In the West, a tantric ritual involving all five taboos includes random sexual coupling. The sexual union itself is accomplished according to strict ritual and with great dignity and meditative visualization. Generally, the purpose of sexual union is the healthy circulation of vital energy between the male and female partners.

Tantrism is neither orgiastic nor hedonistic in principle on the one hand, so to speak, nor is it ascetic. Discipline is essential to Tantric practice. For example, semen is equated with the impulse toward enlightenment and should not be discharged. Orgasm does not lead to bliss but merely to pleasurable sensations. Thus the earnest practitioner must forgo orgasm. Men are advised to apply pressure to the perineum to prevent ejaculation. Some practitioners learn to control their genital functions to the point where they can suck the ejaculated semen back through the penis.

The same consideration applies to women, although in Chinese Taoism, for example, orgasm is not seen to have the same depleting effect as in men. The female sexual secretions, or equivalent of semen, are called *rajas*, which may refer to the hormone-rich vaginal secretions released during sexual arousal. In some schools, men are urged to absorb the female rajas into their own bodies.

In tantra yoga, and yoga in general, sexual activity is not a moral matter, and sexual drive is considered inherently divine. The only reason for suggesting chastity is purely a matter of economics: conservation of energy.

Contemporary applications of yoga as therapy

As age-old traditions of yoga and meditation enter contemporary health care, they represent ways to help manage stress and chronic diseases, and to promote good health. The health benefits of yoga have been proven by scientific research. There is much research on related practices of hypnotherapy, biofeedback, and relaxation techniques, independent of yoga, as well as research specifically associated with yoga. The biofeedback technique in particular has great promise for beginners and for those who are not making discernible progress in meditation, even after constant practice.

The practice of yoga produces physiological changes in the body, as scientifically proven. The monitoring and understanding of these changes have led to a greater understanding of the human body, particularly with regard to the bioenergetic aspects. Basic research has also been done on the psychological aspects of yoga practice. Personal psychology has methods for assessing states of consciousness, and alterations in consciousness through yoga practice have also been shown scientifically. Psychosynthesis, for example, has the same aims as yoga: integration of the whole being of an individual and eventual self-realization. Both modern psychology and yoga emphasize the importance of evolution and growth from "less wholeness" to "more wholeness."

Yoga has been studied as part of contemporary biomedical research in both in India and the West. New scientific research in physiology and psychology has allowed us to gain a better understanding of the human body and mind, and also now forms a body of evidence specifically on complementary medicine as an aid to good health.

Clinical studies have shown that yoga is effective therapy for a range of chronic conditions, as well as for stress management. For example, yoga has been found helpful in the treatment of heart disease and high blood pressure. Yoga is also helpful in the management of asthma and other breathing disorders, and it can improve mood and counter mild depression.

A number of musculoskeletal disorders and common occupational health problems may be managed with yoga, such as carpal tunnel syndrome, osteoarthritis, and low back pain. Preliminary evidence indicates that yoga may also be helpful in disorders of the immune system, such as rheumatoid arthritis and lupus. Yoga and meditation have also been seen to improve academic and physical performance in schoolchildren, potentially contributing to healthy growth and development.

One of the most important changes that take place in the body during meditation and yoga is the slowing down of the metabolism, resulting in a sharp reduction in oxygen consumption and carbon dioxide output by up to 20 percent. Although blood pressure and heart rate decrease overall, peripheral blood flow increases during meditation; activities of the sympathetic nervous system are reduced, and constriction of the blood vessels is decreased. This peripheral blood flow ensures that oxygen is more efficiently delivered to the muscles and that lactate is more quickly and effectively removed. Reduction of lactate level has a direct effect on reduction of blood pressure and anxiety levels.

The quality of relaxation produced by yoga and meditation may be deeper than that produced by sleep, allowing recuperation of the body from the damaging effects of overproduction of adrenaline and activity of the sympathetic nervous system. Through meditation, the septal region of the limbic system in the base of the brain may become operational for the predominant part of our lives. Ideally, proper activation of the brain leads to a life of relaxation, which at the same time, is more efficient and disease free.

Yoga practice involves the total body and total mind. Yoga and meditation act as a holistic treatment concerning the whole mind-body complex. Yoga provides a powerful way of controlling physiological processes and also of controlling physiological reactions to psychological events.

Heart connection

In yoga, individual consciousness is thought to be connected with the physical body at the heart. This consciousness, in an unenlightened individual, is labeled "self-contraction." This contraction is felt at the level of the heart as a sense of separation, isolation, loneliness, fear, and uncertainty. At the level of the mind, this contraction manifests itself as doubt. Yoga endeavors to expand this contraction.

In the West, yoga often is reduced to fitness training bereft of the consciousness and spirit that can be brought to heart and mind. Although reductionist yoga practice helps many people maintain and restore physical health, it does not provide the full potential benefits of yoga. Many practitioners of yoga, in India as well as the West, know only this reductionist form of yoga.

Yoga was never intended for quick fixes or as a cheap service to the ego. Promises of enlightenment over a weekend or a week are misconceptions. Like anything in life, the benefits from yoga are commensurate with the attention, discipline, and effort put into it. Yoga must be learned from a knowledgeable master. A mature student will have no difficulty in learning from a master in any given field. We must, however, examine our teachers carefully. As proven constantly in our daily experience, neither education nor age is any guarantee of wisdom. The mass media have profitably manipulated public opinion by confusing the guru tradition with the vexing issues of cult leadership and brainwashing. As more flamboyant and questionable gurus are replaced through experience with true spiritual masters, the maturing practice of yoga should gain in strength as a means of undertaking the journey from body to spirit.

Chapter 6

Quantum Healing

Maharishi Ayurveda

Maharishi Ayurveda provides a living, breathing example of India's healing traditions. During centuries of foreign rule, the great Ayurvedic institutions of India declined or were actively suppressed, and much of the Ayurvedic knowledge was fragmented, misunderstood, and not used in its totality. The latter part of the twentieth century witnessed an active effort to restore Ayurveda in its wholeness, in accordance with the classical texts, by Maharishi Mahesh Yogi, in collaboration with leading Ayurvedic scholars and physicians, known as vaidyas. Maharishi Ayurveda (MAV) is not only a restoration, but also a reincarnation of the ancient tradition incorporating the insights of the modern physics of quantum mechanics (see Chapters 1 and 2).

What's in the name?

The Sanskrit name Ayurveda is a compound of two words: Ayus, which means "life" or "life span," and Veda, which means whole or complete "knowledge." These ancient terms taken together have been interpreted as the "science of life," or the "science of longevity." The element of "wholeness" in

Ayurvedic knowledge has profound health significance: MAV now encompasses more than twenty treatment approaches dealing with a full range of human life experience: the mind, body, behavior, environment, and, importantly, consciousness, or the "inner life."

MAV considers consciousness to be of primary importance in maintaining optimal health, and emphasizes meditation techniques to foster integrated (holistic) functioning of the nervous system.

MAV includes a sophisticated theoretical framework that provides insight into the functioning of mind and body together.

Understanding of mind-body type is essential to diagnosis and treatment.

Emphasis is placed on the therapeutic effects of diet and healthy digestion, as well as techniques to balance behavior and emotions.

An extensive *materia medica* describes the therapeutic use of medicinal plants.

There is a detailed understanding of biological rhythms, which form the basis for daily and seasonal behavioral routines to strengthen the immune system and homeostatic mechanisms.

Classics of healing

Ancient Ayurvedic texts typically begin with a thorough description of strategies of prevention before discussing modalities for treatment. The Ayurvedic Classics include three major texts (*Brihat Trayi*), the *Charaka Samhita, Sushruta Samhita*, and *Ashtanga Hridaya of Vagbhata*, and three minor texts (*Laghu Trayi*), the *Sarngadhara Samhita, Bhavaprakash Samhita*, and *Madhava Nidanam*. Most of these texts have been translated into English.

These texts address eight main sections of Ayurveda:

- *Kaya Chikitsa*: treatment, diagnosis, and internal medicine.

- *Kaumarya Birtya*: pediatrics, obstetrics, and gynecology.

- *Agad Tantra*: toxicology and medical jurisprudence.

- *Bhut Vidya*: psychosomatic medicine.

- *Rasayana*: *materia medica* to promote vitality, stamina, resistance to disease, and longevity.

- *Vajikarana*: fertility and potency.

- *Shalya*: general surgery.

- *Shalakya*: head and neck surgery.

It is interesting to note that among ancient Egyptian medical texts dating to similarly great antiquity, such as the Edwin Smith papyrus, surgery of the head and neck is also treated separately (see Chapter 3). Further, the Egyptians also qualified medical conditions as "diseases I will treat," "diseases with which I will contend," and essentially incurable diseases.

Worldwide reach

MAV is being practiced in clinics worldwide in India, Europe, Japan, Africa, Russia, Australia, and South and North America by specially trained physicians. In various ways, MAV directs its objectives not only to individual patients, but also to the life of society as a whole. Western biomedicine bases its model for understanding health and disease on the material of the body, while Maharishi Ayurveda is based on the body's non-material essence, which is conceived as a field of pure intelligence. Western medicine's paradigm may seem to be more "scientific," but in certain respects, Ayurveda's model may better encompass today's advanced theories of physics.

Vedic field

We touch on physics again (see Chapter 1) to understand the most basic application of the consciousness model of Maharishi Ayurveda. Vedic thought discusses a unified field of pure, non-material intelligence and consciousness whose modes of vibration manifest as the material universe. These modes of vibration are called Veda. They are described in the voluminous Vedic literature. The Vedic description is strikingly similar to that of physics and emphasizes a key idea that the unified field is the field of pure consciousness. The differentiation between consciousness and matter, between knower and known, loses its significance at the level of the unified field. The different aspects of Vedic literature have been found to correspond with different areas of the physiology (Nader 2000).

In Maharishi Ayurveda, the ultimate basis of disease is losing one's connection to (or, to use a central Vedic description, one's *memory* of) the unified field, which is the innermost core of one's own being and experience. (Samuel Johnson (1709–1784), a seventeenth-century British philosopher of the Age of Reason, stated that "people need to be reminded more often than they need to be instructed.")

This *memory loss* is known as pragya-aparadh. The ultimate basis of prevention and cure is restoring one's conscious connection to (or memory of) this innermost core of one's being and experience. This reconnection, or restoration of memory, is the basis of an integrated approach to health care. Integration of the different layers of life begins with reconnecting one's life to the substrate of all its layers. The innermost core of one's experience is considered identical to the core of all the laws of nature that operate throughout the universe. The body contains, at its basis, the total potential of natural law (just as our DNA contains the total potential of all of our cells in each cell). Maharishi Ayurveda's modalities aim to enable the full expression of the body's inner intelligence. This intriguing possibility is given expression through the idea of Transcendental Consciousness and the practice of Transcendental Meditation, together with other modalities of MAV.

Transcendental meditation and MAV modalities

Means for accomplishing restoration of the body's memory are provided by Vedic techniques for developing consciousness, the most important of which is Transcendental Meditation (TM). The term transcendental indicates that the mind transcends even the subtlest impulses of thought and settles down to the simplest state of awareness (in MAV terms, identical to the unified field). This state of awareness is known technically as Transcendental Consciousness (TC).

During the subjective experience of TC, the metabolism and electroencephalogram (EEG) take on a unique pattern of profound physiological rest and balance, with a metabolic reduction significantly deeper than that experienced during sleep or eyes-closed rest (Wallace 1970). Somewhat paradoxically, with this metabolic rest, blood flow to the brain increases markedly (Jevning *et al.* 1996). The brain displays a state of "restful alertness," characterized by greatly increased coherence between the EEG patterns of different areas of the brain, that is, stable phase relations between two EEG signals as measured by Fourier analyses that attain correlations of more than 0.95 (Badawi *et al.* 1984; Levine 1976). The state of TC can thus be defined physiologically and experientially. This state can be seen to corroborate Maharishi Ayurveda's view of TC as a fourth state of consciousness, in that the three common states of waking, sleeping, and dreaming are distinctly defined physiologically.

With time, the regular practice of the TM technique results in increased coherence that is experienced not only during the meditative process but also during daily activities. Long-term TM practitioners have significantly higher values of frontal EEG coherence during computer tasks compared to subjects who do not practice TM (Travis and Arenander 2006). A study on college students revealed significant brain wave differences between eyes-closed rest and TM practice in EEG coherence, power, and eLORETA cortical activation patterns. These findings indicate that the practice of TM may lead to a foundational state of cerebral functioning that may underlie more focused cognitive processes (Travis *et al.* 2010).

Maharishi Ayurveda views the unfolding of consciousness as the most important strategy for prevention and cure. Consistent with this theory, data suggest that the regular experience of TC has significant health benefits. Such research supports the MAV concept that "remembering" the unified field enlivens the orderly patterns that prevail in a healthy body. For example, TM has been found in several studies to slow biological aging by certain measures (Wallace *et al.* 1982). A study at Harvard of elderly nursing home residents compared TM with two other types of meditation and relaxation techniques over three years.

The TM group had the lowest mortality rate and the greatest reductions in stress and blood pressure (Alexander *et al.* 1989).

A recent meta-analysis of nine randomized controlled trials indicated that the regular practice of TM is associated with a significant reduction in systolic and diastolic blood pressure (Anderson, Liu and Kryscio 2008). TM has been shown to reduce cholesterol (Cooper and Aygen 1978, 1979) and lipid peroxide levels (Schneider *et al.* 1998). A non-invasive method of detecting free radical activity indicates that TM practitioners have lower levels of free radical activity compared to controls who do not meditate (Van Wijk *et al.* 2006). A study on catecholamine levels in TM practitioners showed that epinephrine and norepinephrine levels were significantly lower in the TM group compared with the control group, indicating that the regular practice of TM results in a low hormonal response to daily stress (Infante *et al.* 2001). A randomized controlled clinical trial showed that TM is associated with a reduction in atherosclerosis (Castillo-Richmond *et al.* 2000). A randomized controlled study of African Americans with congestive heart failure showed that TM significantly improved functional capacity (Jayadevappa *et al.* 2007).

A meta-analysis of research on meditation conducted at the Stanford Research Institute found TM to be approximately twice as effective as other meditation techniques in reducing anxiety (Eppley, Abrams and Shear 1989). Orme-Johnson and Walton (1998) conducted an analysis of meditation and relaxation techniques that showed TM to be more effective than other approaches in reducing anxiety, improving psychological health, and reducing tobacco, alcohol, and drug use.

These and similar studies and meta-analyses (Alexander *et al.* 1994a) seem to corroborate Maharishi Ayurveda's theory that simple relaxation or meditation appeared to be not as significant a variable as experiencing the fourth state of consciousness: Transcendental Consciousness. Hundreds of other published studies on TM have for the past few decades documented a wide range of benefits in such areas as intellectual development and rehabilitation (Chalmers *et al.* 1989a, 1989b, 1989c; Orme-Johnson and Farrow 1977; Wallace *et al.* 1989).

Regular practice of TM has also been found to reduce health care costs significantly, as measured by insurance statistics; TM practitioners needed hospitalization for illness or surgery 80 percent less often than a matched control group (Orme-Johnson 1987). A study of Canadian citizens over the age of 65 enrolled in the government health insurance program showed that practice of the TM technique reduced mean government payments to physicians by 24 percent annually compared to controls. There was a five-year cumulative decline of 70 percent in physician payments compared to controls (Herron and Cavanaugh 2005). This suggests that the TM program would be a valuable component of any comprehensive healthcare cost containment strategy or healthcare system reform effort.

Three constitutions and four states of consciousness

Seeing the body as a *pattern of intelligence* is the basis of a central tenet of MAV that it is necessary to maintain the body's natural state of internal balance for optimal health. This tenet has applications for strengthening immunity, as well as for prevention, diagnosis, and treatment. The natural state of balance is understood in terms of another important Ayurvedic concept: three constitutional principles known as doshas govern the functioning of the body, as we have seen in Chapter 3 on Traditional Ayurveda.

However, in light of contemporary quantum science, the three doshas can be more clearly seen to have energetic significance. The three doshas of vata, pitta, and kapha have specific qualities and govern certain physiological activities. The doshas are not thought of as specifically physiological, but rather as subtle principles that emerge early in the manifestation of the unified field. Therefore, they are understood to operate throughout nature.

Of the doshas, vata governs flow and motion in the body. It is at the basis of the activity of the locomotor system. Vata controls functions such as blood circulation, the expansion and contraction of the lungs and heart, intestinal peristalsis and elimination, activities of the nervous system, the contractile process in muscle, ionic transport across membranes (e.g., the sodium pump), cell division, and unwinding of DNA during the process of transcription or replication. Vata is of prime importance in all homeostatic mechanisms and controls the other two principles, pitta and kapha.

Pitta governs bodily functions concerned with heat and metabolism, and directs all biochemical reactions and the process of energy exchange. For example, it regulates digestion, functions of the exocrine glands and endocrine hormones, and intracellular metabolic pathways such as glycolysis, the tricarboxylic acid cycle, and the respiratory chain.

Kapha governs the structure and cohesion of the organism. It is responsible for biological strength, natural tissue resistance, and proper body structure. Microscopically, it is related to anatomical connections in the cell, such as the intracellular matrix, cell membrane, membranes of organelles, and synapses. On a biochemical level, kapha structures receptors and the various forms of chemical binding.

When the doshas are balanced in their natural states and bodily locations, they produce health; when aggravated or imbalanced, they produce disease. A balanced pitta dosha, for example, ensures healthy digestion, while an aggravated pitta can cause acid indigestion and ulcers. MAV holds that all disease results from disruption of the natural balance of the doshas, and immune strength results from maintaining balance of the doshas. The natural dosha balance can be thrown off by a wide variety of factors, such as unhealthy diet, poor digestion, unnatural daily routine, pollutants, and certain behaviors. The balance is restored by a variety of dietary and behavioral modalities, as well as other modalities discussed in this chapter, such as TM and herbal preparations.

The concept of doshas—underlying metabolic principles—simplifies the healthcare practitioner's tasks and increases his or her effectiveness. The tridosha concept can help in clarifying the possible side effects of any treatment, customizing treatments for a specific patient, predicting risk factors and tendencies toward specific diseases, and noticing clusters of apparently unrelated symptoms that may be linked to similar underlying causes.

Doshas, disorders and diseases

The doshas have the ability to provide a basis for more precise description of the individual's natural state of balance. An individual may have a natural predominance of one or more doshas. These doshas need not be present in equal proportion to ensure physiological balance, but they need to be functioning in harmony with one another. This state is called prakriti. When the doshas are out of balance, they create vikriti, resulting in disorder and disease. Table 6.1 describes the classic characteristics of vata, pitta, and kapha prakritis. More common than these are mixed prakritis, which involve various combinations of the three classic types, such as vata-pitta, or pitta-kapha, also describing the normal state of balance for individuals who possess them. Treatment is tailored to the individual patient through careful

Table 6.1 Vata, pitta, and kapha

Vata (ectomorphic constitution)	Pitta (mesomorphic constitution)	Kapha (endomorphic constitution)
Light, thin build	Moderate build	Solid, heavier build
Performs activity quickly	Performs activity with medium speed	Greater strength and endurance
Tendency to dry skin	Aversion to hot weather	Slow, methodical in activity
Aversion to cold weather	Sharp hunger and digestion	Oily, smooth skin
Irregular hunger and digestion	Medium time to grasp new information	Tranquil, steady personality
Quick to grasp new information, also quick to forget	Medium memory	Slow to grasp new information, slow to forget
Tendency toward worry	Tendency toward irritability and temper	Slow to become excited or irritated
Tendency toward constipation	Enterprising and sharp in character	Sleep is heavy and for long periods
Tendency toward light and interrupted sleep	Prefers cold foods and drinks	Hair is plentiful, tends to be dark color
	Cannot skip meals	Slow digestion, mild hunger
	Good speakers	
	Tendency toward reddish complexion and hair, moles, and freckles	

evaluation of both prakriti and vikriti. A pilot study revealed the possibility of utilizing prakriti to correlate phenotypes with genotypes in the human population, which could have wide-ranging implications for health care (Patwardhan, Joshi and Chopra 2005).

Maharishi Ayurveda views disease as resulting from disruption of the natural balance of the doshas, and these doshas accordingly play a key role in MAV's approach to understanding disease. In Western medicine a disease is detected as a result of its symptoms. The emergence of symptoms, however, must be preceded by earlier stages of imbalance in which the body is trying to adapt, or maintain homeostasis, without yet producing frank disease abnormalities in the cells and tissues of the body. The common functional complaints of modern society such as headaches, fatigue, irritable bowel, and pre-menstrual syndromes are disorders occuring at the earlier stages of imbalance before frank pathology is produced. While Western medicine is often impotent in identifying and treating these disorders, a strength of comprehensive, holistic medicine like MAV is addressing problems at this stage before they actually cause irreversible disease.

MAV identifies six stages of pathogenesis, the first three of which have highly subtle symptoms with which allopathic medicine is not familiar. These first three stages essentially involve aggravation of the normal functioning of the doshas. A skilled MAV diagnostician can detect these early pathogenic stages before overt symptoms emerge.

Maharishi Ayurveda uses a number of diagnostic techniques. All of them are non-invasive and reveal much information about underlying imbalances and about specific illnesses. Chief among these techniques is *nadi vigyan* (pulse diagnosis), which allows one to retrieve detailed information about the internal functioning of the body and its organs through signals present in the radial pulse. This information involves not only the cardiovascular system but other bodily systems as well. From the pulse, the diagnostician gains information about the functioning of the bodily tissues, the state of the doshas, and much more. Pulse diagnosis reveals early stages of imbalance that precede full-blown symptoms. In this and other MAV diagnostic modalities, perceiving the body as a pattern of intelligence enables physicians to retrieve enormous amounts of information in a non-invasive manner.

Planted in consciousness

Western pharmacology, applying the mechanistic model of the body, synthesizes single chemicals as active ingredients, or isolates and then synthesizes single active ingredients from herbs and plants. The active-ingredient model reflects a limitation of the scientific method: its inability to deal with complex systems and its requirement that the researcher radically, unnaturally, and unrealistically simplify a biological process in order to evaluate it (Sharma 1997). In contrast, Ayurvedic pharmacology, called *dravyaguna*, uses the synergistic cooperation of substances as they coexist in natural sources. It uses single plants or, more often, mixtures of plants whose effects are complementary. Such synergistic effects are gaining consideration in Western medical research, which is finding, for example, that combinations of antioxidants suppress inflammation (Haines *et al.* 2010) and combinations of chemotherapeutic agents inhibit cancer cell growth (Rosano *et al.* 2010), more effectively than these substances acting alone.

In terms of MAV's consciousness model, the effectiveness of herbal mixtures relative to active ingredients can be explained by the idea that plants, especially herbs, are concentrated repositories of nature's intelligence, which, when used properly, can increase the expression of that intelligence in the body. Research and experience with Maharishi Ayurveda herbal mixtures known as rasayanas shows that synergism enhances, for example, the free radical scavenging properties of herbs and mitigates the harmful side effects that often accompany Western drugs (Sharma 2002).

According to Maharishi Ayurveda, rasayanas promote longevity, stamina, immunity, and overall well-being (Sharma 1993). Research has shown several rasayanas to have significant antioxidant properties (Bondy, Hernandez and Mattia 1994; Cullen *et al.* 1997; Dwivedi *et al.* 1991, 2005; Engineer, Sharma and Dwivedi 1992; Hanna *et al.* 1994; Niwa 1991; Sharma *et al.* 1995). The rasayana known as *Maharishi Amrit Kalash* (MAK) is approximately one thousand times more effective at scavenging free radicals than vitamin C, vitamin E, and a pharmaceutical antioxidant (Sharma *et al.* 1992).

MAK has been researched extensively in laboratory, animal, and clinical settings, and has been found to have a wide range of significant beneficial properties. MAK has prevented and treated breast cancer (Sharma *et al.* 1990; Sharma *et al.* 1991); prevented metastasis of lung cancer (Patel *et al.* 1992); caused nervous system tumor cells (neuroblastoma) to regain normal cell functioning (Prasad *et al.* 1992); enhanced the effect of nerve growth factor in causing morphological differentiation of nervous system tumor cells (pheochromocytoma) (Rodella *et al.* 2004); inhibited the growth of skin cancer cells (melanoma) (Prasad, Parry and Chan 1993); and inhibited liver cancer (Penza *et al.* 2007). In clinical studies, MAK has been shown to reduce the side effects of chemotherapy without reducing the efficacy of the cancer treatment (Misra *et al.* 1994; Srivastava *et al.* 2000).

MAK also reduces several risk factors for heart disease. It has prevented human platelet aggregation (Sharma, Feng and Penganamala 1989) and reduced atherosclerosis in laboratory animals by 53 percent (Lee *et al.* 1996). In clinical studies on patients with heart disease, MAK reduced the frequency of angina, improved exercise tolerance, and lowered systolic blood pressure and lipid peroxide levels (Dogra *et al.* 1994; Dogra and Bhargava 2005). A study on hyperlipidemic patients showed that MAK increases the resistance of low-density lipoprotein to oxidation, which is important for the prevention of atherosclerosis (Sundaram *et al.* 1997).

A strong immune system is vital to the maintenance of health. Several studies have shown that MAK significantly enhances immune functioning (Dileepan *et al.* 1990, 1993; Inaba *et al.* 1995, 1996, 1997, 2005). MAK has also demonstrated antiaging effects. It improved age-related visual discrimination in older men (Gelderloos *et al.* 1990) and has been shown to rejuvenate the antioxidant defense system and protect against mitochondrial deterioration in the aging central nervous system (Vohra *et al.* 1999, 2001a). In the aging brain, MAK reduced lipid peroxidation and lipofuscin pigment accumulation, restored normal oxygen consumption, and enhanced cholinergic enzymes (Vohra *et al.* 2001b, 2001c). It has also been shown to decrease the number of dark neurons in the brain, which indicates that MAK protects the neurons from injury (Vohra *et al.* 2002).

A modified form of MAK, known as Amrit Nectar tablets, has powerful antioxidant properties. In a study on the inhibition of lipid peroxidation, the aqueous extract of Amrit Nectar tablets was 16 times more potent and the alcoholic extract was 166 times more potent than vitamin E, a well-known antioxidant. Amrit Nectar tablets also protected against the toxic side effects of the chemotherapeutic drugs doxorubicin (Adriamycin) and cisplatin (Dwivedi *et al.* 2005).

Foods and fundamentals

Western medical research is accumulating increasing evidence that diet plays a critical role in the development of heart disease and cancer. The American Cancer Society reports that about one-third of the cancer deaths that occur each year in the United States have diet as a significant risk factor (American Cancer Society 2010). Scientists estimate that 60 to 70 percent of cancers can be prevented by simple changes in diet and lifestyle. It is known that a diet rich in the wrong types of fat creates a higher risk of heart disease, currently the number one killer in the United States (American Heart Association 2007). Ayurveda has long considered problems of diet and digestion to be among the central causes of all disease and has considered improvement of diet and digestion to be crucial to almost any therapeutic regimen. Ayurveda views faulty diet as not only contributing to specific degenerative diseases, but also throwing off the body's natural balance, thus weakening immunity.

MAV's approach to diet rests on the consciousness model. Food is viewed as providing not only matter and energy to the body but also intelligence, order, and balance. MAV dietetics considers not only the nutritional value and caloric content of food but also the food's impact on the body's underlying state of balance. Foods affect the doshas, and diet must be suited to the individual vikriti and prakriti. It must also reflect the climate and season, as well as specific health conditions. In short it must be in balance with nature and with the individual's natural predispositions.

The influence of food on the doshas is specific to the food, but can usually be determined by knowing in which generic categories of taste and qualities the food belongs. According to MAV, the six categories of taste are sweet, sour, salty, pungent, bitter, and astringent. The major categories of food qualities are heavy, light, oily, dry, hot, and cold. Tastes and food qualities affect the doshas, and different foods possess these various qualities and tastes.

To give an example of how this information would be applied clinically, a patient with kapha syndromes (e.g., sinusitis, certain types of obesity) would be advised to minimize eating heavy, oily, and cold foods, as well as foods with sweet, sour, and salty tastes. It would be recommended that the patient give predominance to foods exhibiting the remaining qualities and tastes.

MAV recommends a lactovegetarian diet for optimal health. Meat is difficult to digest, and has been linked to numerous diseases, including heart disease, cancer (Sinha *et al.* 2009), and diabetes (Vang *et al.* 2008; Song *et al.* 2004). It should also be noted that the nutritional composition of domestic meats (versus wild game) has been radically altered during the past century by changes in animal husbandry, and by the use of antibiotics and synthetics in the raising of livestock for food.

Vegetarian diets, and diets high in fruits and vegetables, have been shown to have protective effects against cancer, whereas eating meat has been correlated with the development of various types of cancer. Non-vegetarians have a significantly higher risk of developing colon cancer and prostate cancer (Fraser 1999). Women who eat red meat daily are at twice the risk of developing colon cancer compared to women who eat red meat less than once a month (Willett *et al.* 1990). A large prospective study, the National Institutes of Health-AARP Diet and Health Study, found that eating red meat is associated with a significantly elevated risk of colorectal cancer, lung cancer, esophageal cancer, and liver cancer. Eating processed meats resulted in a significantly elevated risk of colorectal cancer and lung cancer (Cross *et al.* 2007). A study on vegetarians found over one-third reduction in cancer mortality in the non-meat eaters compared to meat eaters (Thorogood *et al.* 1994). Increased consumption of fruit has been associated with lower risks of lung, prostate, and pancreatic cancers (Fraser 1999).

Multiple studies have demonstrated that increased risk of heart disease is associated with eating meat, whereas a vegetarian diet affords protection against heart disease. A study on Seventh-Day Adventists showed a significant association between beef consumption and fatal ischemic heart disease in men, compared to vegetarians. The lifetime risk of ischemic heart disease was reduced by over one-third in male vegetarians compared to non-vegetarians (Fraser 1999). The risk of developing ischemic heart disease is also significantly lower in older vegetarian women compared with older non-vegetarian women (Kwok *et al.* 2000).

Considering all the benefits of increased consumption of fruits and vegetables in the diet, it is not surprising that studies have shown vegetarians have a longer life span (Fraser 1999). A long-term study found that vegetarians have a mortality rate that is half that of the general population (Key *et al.* 1996).

Diet and digestion

Maharishi Ayurveda focuses not only on *what one eats* but also on *how one digests it*. The emphasis on digestion contrasts with Western allopathic medicine, which deals with digestion only when it becomes significantly disrupted. In MAV, excellent digestion is considered critical to robust health. MAV contains a number of techniques for improving digestion and treating digestive disorders. They center on the concept of agni, which literally means "fire," and refers to metabolic and digestive activities that convert foodstuff into bodily substances. Ayurveda describes 13 types of agni in the body. Their importance in Ayurvedic health care is suggested by the fact that one of the eight branches of Ayurveda, Kaya Chikitsa (internal medicine), focuses on the strength or weakness of the agnis. This emphasis on digestion becomes clear when considering the end product of poor digestion, which Ayurveda calls ama. Ama can be understood as accumulated toxic substances at different levels of the physiology. At the level of gross digestion, poorly-digested food results in a thick, slimy material that lines the walls of the bowel, impeding absorption and assimilation of nutrients. At the cellular level, during functioning of the physiology there is accumulation of impurities and toxins. These impurities come from both inside and outside the body. From inside the body come internal metabolic and cellular waste products, such as free radical-damaged cells and tissues, and from outside come external impurities and toxins, such as pollutants and toxins that occur naturally in food. All these impurities are collectively referred to as ama in Vedic terminology (Sharma 2004). Ama plays a key role in pathogenesis, interacting with aggravated doshas and causing them to "stick" to areas where they do not belong. Healthy digestion reduces the amount of ama produced.

The central role of food and digestion is demonstrated particularly well by consideration of another central MAV concept: the importance of a substance called ojas. Ojas is said to be the finest manifestation of the unified field, which serves as a sort of glue to link consciousness and matter. Ojas is the master coordinator between consciousness and the physiology, and mind and body.

Ojas maintains the integrity of the seven fundamental principles that support the various bodily tissues (*dhatus*) which are: plasma (*rasa*), blood (*rakta*), muscle (*mamsa*), fat (*meda*), bone (*asthi*), bone marrow and nervous system (*majja*), and sperm/ovum (*sukra*). Ojas promotes balanced growth in the body and enhances the immune system. The end product of truly healthy diet and digestion is said to contain significant amounts of ojas. According to an MAV expression, "Like a bee that gets honey from the flowers, we get ojas from our food." Most MAV therapies and behavioral advice are designed to maximize the presence of ojas, and almost all MAV proscriptions are designed to minimize the depletion of ojas.

The manner in which food is eaten is considered to have an effect on healthy digestion. Food should be eaten in a warm, congenial, and uplifting atmosphere. Arguing or any other negativity at meals interferes with digestion, producing ama instead of ojas. Positive, loving emotions enhance digestion and increase the abundance of ojas. The importance of eating in convivial circumstances is underscored by the emphasis on community and family meals in "old world" Western culture as well. Looking beyond what is eaten, the importance of how we eat is demonstrated by the Italian-American community of Roseto, near Scranton PA, where people eat all the "wrong" foods but under the right circumstances. They have half the heart disease rates that would otherwise be predicted by diet alone. In Europe, the "French Paradox" consistently demonstrates half the rates of chronic diseases compared to the United States despite the consumption of more rich foods, more tobacco and more wine. But the French take more time with their meals, both preparation and consumption, and emphasize a more relaxed lifestyle.

De-tox and purification

To rid the body of accumulated ama, pollutants, and other pathogenic and undigested impurities that disrupt or block the natural expression of the body's inner intelligence, Maharishi Ayurveda emphasizes the importance of purification therapies. Foremost among these is *Panchakarma* (or Pañchakarma), which literally means "five activities." Panchakarma includes five main treatment modalities:

1. Whole-body massage with herbalized oil (*abhyanga*).

2. Continuous flow of warm herbalized oil on the forehead (*shirodhara*).

3. Fomentation of the body with herbalized heat (*swedana*).

4. Special herbalized oil head massage and nasal administration of herbs (*nasya*).

5. Sesame oil retention or herbalized eliminative enemas (*basti*).

Daily treatments, administered for one week or longer, are recommended with each change of the seasons. Certain aspects of Panchakarma can also fit easily into a patient's daily preventive regimen. Preliminary research has shown that regular Panchakarma reduces several cardiovascular risk factors, including cholesterol (Sharma 1993; Waldschütz 1988). Sesame oil, which is typically used for colonic irrigation in Panchakarma, has been shown to inhibit in vitro malignant melanoma growth (Smith and Salerno 1992) and human colon adenocarcinoma cell line growth (Salerno and Smith 1991). Preliminary research on Panchakarma has shown that it reduces fat-soluble toxicants in humans. Levels of polychlorinated biphenyls (PCBs) and agrochemicals were reduced by 50 percent in subjects who received Panchakarma. PCBs have been banned for years, but previous exposure can result in a lingering accumulation of the toxicant in fat tissue. Lipophilic toxicants have been associated with hormonal disorders, suppression of the immune system, reproductive disorders, cancer, and other diseases (Herron and Fagan 2002).

See no evil, hear no evil, speak no evil

A symbol of ancient Asian philosophy is provided by the three primates, depicted with hands folded over eyes, ears and mouth: "see no evil, hear no evil, speak no evil" expressed in traditional art and religion. These ancient virtues are reflected in the healthy functioning of the body, and are stressed as important social mores.

Maharishi Ayurveda regards behavior, speech, and emotions as having a significant impact on health. This concept springs naturally from the model that places consciousness at the basis of the body. Emotions can be understood as fine fluctuations of consciousness (or the unified field); as such, their impact on the more expressed physical levels of the body are immense. Ayurvedic texts include detailed discussions of lifestyle and behavior and their impact on health. Interestingly, traditional virtues—such as respect for elders, teachers, loved ones, and family members; pardoning those who wrong you; practicing nonviolence; and not speaking ill of others—are understood to promote health for the individual's mind and body, as well as for the community and society.

According to Ayurveda, information entering through the five senses (sight, sound, taste, touch, and smell) is digested and metabolized in its own specific ways and the byproducts influence the physiology. Thus, sensory input is considered to have an impact on health. This idea is applied clinically, not only in terms of behavioral advice but also in the form of sensory therapies such as aromatherapy and sound therapy.

Circadian cycles

In Maharishi Ayurveda, attuning the lifestyle to natural biorhythms is considered a crucial element of prevention and treatment. MAV gives a detailed analysis of circadian and circannual rhythms, with recommendations for daily and seasonal routines. These recommendations include rising and retiring early, and eating one's main meal at lunchtime when the digestive "fires" are strongest. Many other recommendations are also given; as always, this advice must be tailored to the individual. Emerging Western data on biorhythms correlate well with ancient Ayurvedic knowledge. Again, the idea of a connection between patterns of order in nature and in the human body seems inherently obvious, or self-evident truth.

The three-dosha concept plays a key role in understanding these connections. Different times of the day are associated with different doshas, as are different seasons and the different stages of the human life cycle (Table 6.2). With regard to the seasons, the dosha predominance varies depending on climatic conditions and geographic location, so it will not be the same in every region of the world. In the United States, vata accumulates when the weather is cold, dry, and windy. Pitta accumulates when the weather is hot. Kapha accumulates when the weather is cold and wet. Vata, pitta, and kapha generally increase during the following seasons:

- vata in late autumn and winter (mid-October to mid-March)

- pitta in summer and early autumn (mid-June to mid-October)

- kapha in spring (mid-March to mid-June).

During the seasons of life, childhood is dominated by kapha (which governs structure, substance, and growth), middle age (time of dynamic activity) by pitta, and old age by vata.

Ayurveda as modern healthcare

In terms of chronic disease, Western medicine has now recognized that preventing diseases and disorders requires changes in lifestyle, diet, and behavior. However, allopathic medicine remains limited as to how to effect these changes in patients for a prolonged time. Research has shown that those who practice TM are better able to give up harmful habits such as cigarette smoking, alcohol consumption, and illegal drug use, and incorporate healthy dietary and lifestyle changes (Alexander, Robinson and Rainforth 1994b).

MAV offers other time-tested modalities that benefit individual patients, such as daily routine and purification procedures, which could be useful in large-scale applications. MAV also offers an overall theory of prevention involving such elements as the three-dosha concept, that could be of value for research on preventive medicine.

Many central elements of Ayurveda, such as the ideas that diet and emotions play a crucial role in disease and prevention, were not taken seriously by Western medicine a generation ago but are now major themes of research. Other areas of Ayurveda might prove to be of value both in clinical practice and research. Already, the Transcendental Meditation technique and herbal preparations have produced bodies of significant research findings whose implications have yet to be fully explored. The clinical use of Ayurveda appears to be most dramatic when applied to diseases that Western medicine finds difficult to treat, such as poor digestion, heart disease, cancer, and other chronic diseases (Janssen 1989).

Table 6.2 Times of day, seasons, and human life cycle

	Vata	**Pitta**	**Kapha**
Time	Approximately 2 a.m. to 6 am (sunrise) and 2 p.m. to 6 p.m.	Approximately 10 a.m. to 2 p.m. and 10 p.m. to 2 a.m.	Approximately 6 a.m. (sunrise) to 10 a.m. and 6 p.m. to 10 p.m.
Season	In Europe and USA, late autumn and winter In India, summer and rainy season	In Europe and USA, summer and early autumn In India, rainy season and autumn	In Europe and USA, spring In India, late winter and spring
Period in life cycle	Old age	Adulthood	Childhood

Ayurveda is a comprehensive system of health care that utilizes multiple modalities for treatment of disorders. Several medical institutions have incorporated Ayurveda into their teaching curricula. In the future it is likely that Ayurveda will gain further recognition as an effective system of natural health care. Its comprehensive modalities can be used to create health and well-being in the individual and in society as a whole. It is a good example of India's living traditions as it grows and adapts with knowledge of modern physics, modern physicians and modern medicine, while maintaining its ancient wisdom about human health and healing.

See the Appendix at the end of the book for Ayurvedic secrets to health and longevity.

Chapter 7

Tibetan Medicine

To the High Himalaya

The Tibetan system of medicine, the science of healing, also has a pedigree of concepts and practices dating back through the centuries. As with many aspects of Tibetan cultural practices, the Tibetan medical system displays a creative mixture of aspects of traditions from the Middle and East Asian regions with those of its varied indigenous practices. Deeply rooted in the cosmology of Buddhism, Tibetan medicine is organized primarily around concepts of the body that are shared with Ayurveda (India's science of life). Tibetan medicine has a classic literature (since the eighth century CE), diverse practices, specialized knowledge, and regional variations.Tibetan medicine shows great adaptability, perhaps greatly due to its links to Buddhism, and the constant reminder that compassion is fundamental to the practice of medicine.

Shaped by mountains

The circumstances that shaped Tibetan medicine are largely the circumstances of geopolitical factors and the unique geography of the Tibetan plateau in the Himalayan Mountains high above the riverine plains of India.

Tibet is isolated both by mountain ranges that surround it on three sides, and by its own geological elevation—the capital of Tibet, Lhasa, stands at nearly 12,000 feet above sea level. The southern border of Tibet is formed by the Himalayan Mountains with Bhutan, Nepal, and India to the south. The Tibetan plateau rises as one moves north. The Kun Lun and the Dang La mountains form a northern border, and beyond them lie Mongolia and China. The Karakoram and Ladakh mountains are to the west, as one moves toward Pakistan and Afghanistan. The eastern border is formed by the Mekong and Salween rivers as they flow from the north and ultimately form deep gorges through Burma to the southeast, with the Salween traversing the course of Burma, and the Mekong traveling eastward to form the borders between Thailand and Laos, then passing through Vietnam, with the massive Mekong Delta comprising a large part of the former South Vietnam. Tibet is surrounded on all sides by challenging landscapes that present immense natural barriers.

At the crossroads of civilization

Tibet lies to the south of the ancient trade route known as the "Silk Road." From at least the second century BCE to the thirteenth century CE, when it began to be outmoded by the merchant sea routes of Greater China, the Silk Road allowed such high-value goods as silk and spices (including medicinal foods and herbs) to be traded all along its length. Precious medicinal plants, such as rhubarb, found their way west to Ancient Greece and Rome. This trade route also furnished conduits for exchange of knowledge and ideas between East and West. The volume of trade along its length fluctuated, depending on geopolitical stability and the security afforded its travelers by local rulers.

During China's Tang Dynasty (618–907 CE), the route was important as a link between the West of the Dark Ages and the cosmopolitan East. Ch'ang-an (just northwest of modern Xian), the famous walled city, was the western terminus of the Silk Road for the Chinese. By the eighth century it was a huge city of almost 2 million. A census completed in 754 CE (shortly after the appearance of Islam in the deserts of Arabia and the Middle

East) documented some five thousand foreigners in the city, including Turks, Iranians, and Indians who had traveled east to come to this trading center.

It is important to recognize that in the absence of any more rapid form of communication, these trading centers and the individuals who moved between them were the sole conduits for the transmission of information as well as goods. Travelers, religious pilgrims, and physicians would exchange knowledge and further enhance the cosmopolitan character of this region.

Rise of the real kings

South of this cultural nexus, Tibet comprised settled communities under the rule of minor princes or feudal lords, as well as dispersed bands of nomadic pastoralists. Although little is known of Tibet before the sixth century CE, tradition holds that a lineage of thirty-one semi-mythical kings, or rulers, preceded this period.

The thirty-second king of Tibet, Namri Songtsen (c. 570–619), in the early seventh century, secured the loyalty of warriors in his region. He consolidated power by gathering the disparate clans of skilled riders into a mobile force that could swiftly shift military force into surrounding territories. Under the reign of his son, the thirty-third king, Songtsen Gampo (c. 609–649), Tibet began expansion. Building on the military successes of his father, Gampo's forces threatened Xian in China and compelled the Tang emperor Tai Zong to grant him a Chinese princess in marriage—securing peace by creating family relationships. Gampo's incursions to the south resulted in his marriage to a Nepalese princess, with the same peace-making result. These two wives are associated with bringing some of the first Buddhist texts to Tibet, and guiding the king toward establishing Buddhism as the state religion.

Languages of healing

At this same time, a written alphabet designed for the Tibetan language was developed, which helped facilitate the translation and transliteration of Sanskrit texts. This commitment to Sanskrit represented a distinct cultural separation between Tibet and China. Although Tibetans showed ongoing interest in Chinese texts, the linguistic commitment to India was an important sign of the cultural orientation intended for Tibet by its ruler. From thenceforth, medical scholars in Tibet had a language in which to record their own knowledge, as well as that obtained from other lands.

The first conference of learned physicians

The focus on India was not exclusive, as King Songtsen Gampo's Chinese wife brought with her a medical text, *Great Analytical Treatise on Medicine*. In addition, Songtsen Gampo sent messengers out across the region (and along the Silk Road) to summon expert physicians to what is now known as the first conference of learned physicians. Three doctors came to Tibet, from India, China, and Persia. Each of the invited physicians brought texts that were then translated into Tibetan. It is said that Galenos, the Persian physician, remained at the Tibetan court, and fathered three sons, who carried his medical lineage to different parts of Tibet.

Following the fall of Rome in the fifth century, the vitality of Greco-Roman culture was isolated in Byzantium. Persian and Arabian physicians explored the wealth of Greco-Roman medical knowledge from such figures as Galen and Dioscorides that was preserved within Byzantium (and Alexandria, Egypt) to incorporate it into their own cultures. Galenos, the Persian physician who adopted his name from Galen, became an exponent of what is known as Unani Tibb, or "Greek" medicine (see Chapter 8).

With the knowledge of the Galenic traditions moving toward Asia from the West, with contact with the East Asian traditions through Xian, China, to the north, and with the profound and privileged influence of Indian culture and medicine from the south, the consummately cosmopolitan character of the Tibetan medical tradition began to be established.

The second conference of learned physicians

By the eighth century, as Tibet continued to exercise its influence throughout the region, its thirty-seventh king came to the throne. Trisong Detsen (c. 741–798 CE) convened the second conference of learned physicians, and the "Four Tantras" were translated and brought to Tibet from India. The king sent messengers out with gifts to bring more physicians from India, Kashmir, China, Persia, Guge (a nearby kingdom), and Nepal. The conferences of learned physicians were opportunities to share knowledge and demonstrate medical acumen. According to one famous version of the events, a patient was placed behind a drawn curtain, and a thin string was wrapped around her wrist and then pulled out through an opening in the curtain. When the string was pulled tight, the vibration of her pulse could be felt through it. Each of the visiting physicians was asked to pull the string taut and to make a diagnosis based on the vibration of the pulse alone, without examining the patient.

Influence of the Four Tantras

While practical skills of diverse physicians were being shared in Tibet, a text arrived in Tibet that would become the basis for the organized study and practice of Tibetan medicine. This text, known as the "Four Tantras," or Gyu She may have been composed in India in about 400 CE. It was both a medical text and a developed expression of the scripture of Northern Buddhism (Mahayana, or the Great Vehicle) in relation to medicine.

The Four Tantras profoundly influenced the Tibetan understanding of medicine. This understanding asserts the primacy of Buddhist medical knowledge, and implies that all healing traditions share the ultimate goal of providing compassionate care to all suffering beings. Because of the importance of Buddhism to the development of Tibetan medicine, it is helpful to have a general understanding of the teachings contained in the Four Tantras and the life of the Buddha.

North with the Buddha

The historical Buddha, Gautama or Sakyamuni, was a privileged prince of the Sakya clan growing up in the sixth century BCE, near what is now Lumbini, Nepal. It is said that as a young man he was struck by a deep, painful awareness that disease, old age, and death are the common fate of all beings. He left his comfortable home, and committed himself to finding a method that would afford release from the suffering that is the innate consequence of living. After years of ascetic practice, he found his way, and awoke to a life that was free of the suffering attendant on the common experiences of birth, disease, old age, and death. When asked by a stranger who he was, Prince Gautama responded to call him "the one who woke up." The "awakened one" (the meaning of the word *Buddha*) then taught others to awaken and free themselves.

The Buddha's teachings persist in the texts and practices of various traditions, originally delivered orally and not recorded in writing until about 100 BCE. Of the major traditions that emerged from Buddha's teachings, the Theravada tradition (which was handed down by "the elders") may be considered more historically based, and was established in India, Sri Lanka, and Southeast Asia, while the Mahayana tradition (which originated the ideal of the *Bodhisattva*, dedicated to freeing all of creation from suffering, earning it the appellation "Great Vehicle") was influential in the development of Buddhism in China, Japan, Mongolia, and Tibet, and may be referred to as "Northern Buddhism." Mahayana scriptures from the first century BCE portray a Buddha whose activities and manifestations transcend those initially attributed to the purely historical figure, Gautama.

The Medicine Buddha

Scriptures state that, during his lifetime, Gautama Buddha manifested the form of the Medicine Buddha (Sanskrit: *Baishajya Guru*) in a celestial palace of medicine, Tanadug. The Medicine Buddha appeared in the form traditionally associated with a peaceful Buddha. His skin is the deep blue of lapis lazuli, and emanates a radiant blue light. In his right hand he holds a branch of myrobalan (*Terminalia chebula*) in the gesture of granting blessings, and in his left hand, which is held in the posture of meditation, he holds a bowl of life-giving nectar. This vivid deity appears in a palace that is surrounded on all sides by medicinal substances.

To the south of the Medicine Buddha lies the mountain known as the "Thunderbolt." It is said to have the power of the sun, and is covered in medicinal plants such as pomegranate, long pepper, and capsicum. These medicines are hot tasting, sour, and salty. They have the qualities of heat and acridity, and thus are said to treat diseases caused by cold. To the north is the "Snow-clad Mountain," which has the power of the moon, and medicines such as sandalwood and camphor grow on it. These medicines are bitter, sweet, and astringent in taste, and have the quality of coolness, thus relieving ailments caused by heat. To the east rises the "Fragrant Mountain," which is covered in a forest of myrobalans. To the west is "Cool Mountain," on which grow medicines such as bamboo, saffron, clove, nutmeg, and cardamoms. It is said that the meadows surrounding the palace are filled with the fragrance of incense, and are inhabited by many animals that provide medicinal substances.

Seated in the center of the palace, the Medicine Buddha is surrounded by Rishis, Buddhists, non-Buddhists, and gods. If you imagine a divine and radiant being seated on a throne in a great palace, surrounded by all the great medicines of Asia and their aromas, and attended by gods, Hindu scholars, sages, and Buddhists, you will capture something of the image conveyed by the Medicine Buddha's mandala (Figure 7.1).

According to this tradition, each group of disciples in attendance on the Medicine Buddha received different teaching according to their dispositions and needs. Rabgay's translation of the text *Ba.Jung.Don.Gong.'Thad* states the following:

> For the sake of beings, the Sugata, through his manifestation, taught the methods of compounding medication in India, moxa and vein clearing in China, and blood letting in Dolpo (now northern Nepal). To the assembly of Gods, he taught the "Verses of Healing," and to the Rishis he taught the "Eight works of Charaka," while to the Non-Buddhists

he taught "Krishna Ishvara Tantra." To the Buddhists he taught "The Teachings of the Three Protectors."

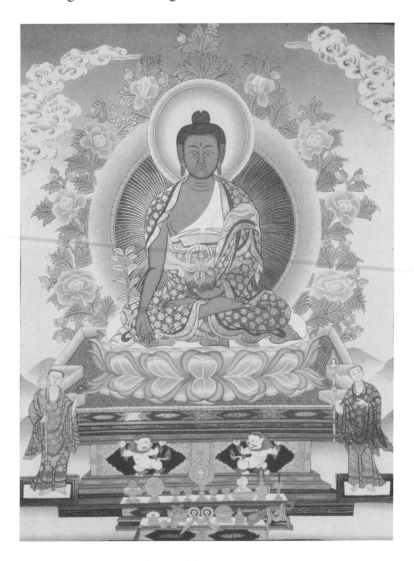

Figure 7.1 The Medicine Buddha's mandala

Within the Buddhist tradition, an enlightened teacher provides information according to the requirements and capabilities of the audience—whether the general public, students, or disciples. Accordingly, medicine was taught within the traditions that reflected the interests of each group.

While teaching according to the propensities of those assembled, the Medicine Buddha simultaneously emanated two divine beings (further manifestations of the Buddha). From his heart appeared the sage Rigpay Yeshe, and from his tongue the sage Yilay Kye. A dialogue ensued, as Yilay Kye posed questions and Rigpay Yeshe answered them. (The dialogue is a traditional form of discourse in Chinese medical classics as well.) This dialogue ultimately became the source of the text, the Four Tantras, that, from at least the twelfth century, exists simultaneously as a sacred text and as a guide to the practice of medicine, describing the fundamentals of the Tibetan approach to healing.

Among all those in attendance, only the sage Yilay Kye heard the teaching of the Four Tantras. According to tradition, these teachings were recorded on gold in lapis lazuli ink and preserved in a sacred realm, the Dakini Palace in Uddiyana. Preserved there by dakinis (feminine agents of wisdom and transformation), the texts were transmitted to the fourth-century author of the Four Tantras as a revealed scripture and, about three centuries later, were translated into Tibetan.

This vivid imagery, as in other scriptures, suggests that we should read these words metaphorically, rather than taking them literally or dismissing them as esoteric. The Medicine Buddha is shown to be providing instruction in every form of medicine in Asia. "Moxa and vein clearing" is essentially the practice of Chinese acupuncture. "Compounding medication" had been a core practice in India for centuries, and the *Caraka Samitha* is one of the most revered texts of Ayurveda.

Primacy of the Buddhist view in medicine

Mahayana Buddhist tradition asserts the mythological primacy of Buddhism even in relation to the sacred origins of Ayurveda. According to Indian mythology, Ayurveda was first perceived (but not written down) by Brahma. He taught this science to Daksa Prajapati, who taught it to the Asvini Kumaras, and they taught it to Indra. The tradition in Tibet explains that Brahma, in fact, simply remembered the teachings on medicine given to him by Kasyapa Buddha. In this manner the antiquity of

Buddhist medical teachings can be asserted, even though the history of Ayurveda precedes that of Gautama Buddha. Similarly, the Mahayana scriptures can be read as establishing the Buddhist roots of every great medical tradition. According to Ergil (2006), given the rivalry and tradition of debate between Buddhist and non-Buddhist schools of thought in India, it is possible to view this claim as a scriptural assertion of primacy (Ergil 2006, p.462). Ergil suggests from the point of view of a Buddhist that every form of medicine contained within the Buddhist healing tradition ultimately is an expression of the Buddha's compassion (Ergil 2006, p.462).

Medicine as a practice in the world

Another feature of the tradition of Northern Buddhism was an emphasis on the possibility of participating in the activities of the world while seeking enlightenment (as can be seen in karma yoga). The early Buddhist scriptures that guided monastic conduct forbade monks from the practice of medicine (prescribing of medicines and minor surgery) as an occupation or means of livelihood. These later scriptures suggest that the application of many of the healing methods of Asia represents the application of the teachings of the Buddha.

The description of the origins of the Four Tantras shows medical systems belonging to other traditions and cultures originating from the Buddha's teachings. This connection establishes the authority and significance of the Buddha as a teacher of medicine. It also expands the range of techniques and traditions that can be included under the heading of "Buddhist medicine." In a similar manner, ascribing the origin of Ayurveda to Kasapya effectively permits all Ayurvedic traditions to be understood as Buddhist medicine.

The Four Tantras

After the Four Tantras came to Tibet during the reign of Trisong Detsen, the thirty-seventh king at the end of the eighth century CE, they were translated by Vairochana, a disciple of Padmasambhava, one of the important teachers of Buddhism in Tibet. Vairochana visited India and received teachings on the Four Tantras from the pandit Candrabhinanda. On his return from India, Vairochana was instructed by his teacher Padmasambhava to hide the text and its translation in a pillar at Samye Monastery. The elder Yuthog Yontan Gonpo (708–833 CE), who was among the court physicians at this time, wrote eighteen supplements to it, and is also credited with the founding of Tanadug Medical College in Kongpo Menlung, said to be the first medical school established in Tibet.

A comprehensive revision of the Four Tantras was carried out by the younger Yuthog Yontan Gonpo (1112–1203 CE). The actual title of the text generally referred to as the "Four Tantras" is *The Ambrosia Heart Tantra: The Secret Oral Teaching on the Eight Branches of the Science of Healing*. This text also guided and informed the medical practices of neighboring Buddhist cultures, such as Mongolia, Ladakh, Sikkim, and Bhutan.

The peace dividend

With the gradual growth of Buddhism, Tibetan interest in military campaigns ended. After a number of royal assassinations during the ninth century, the line of Songtsen Gampo ended. Tibet became a collection of principalities. Lamas (religious teachers) were often given support by the princes, achieving a measure of secular authority. This state of affairs was subsequently altered by a series of relationships between the Mongolian khans and various lamas, which began with an attempt to avoid invasion of Tibet by Chingis Khan in 1107 CE. These relationships added a new element to the competition for secular power between lamas and their Tibetan patron princes. Finally, in 1642, the Fifth Dalai Lama, Ngawang Lobzang Gyatso, was established as the religious head of Tibet by Gusri Khan. By having a holy and reincarnating ruler with a firm grasp on the country, Tibet emerged as a theocratic state with an operational division between secular and religious authorities. The reign of the Fifth Dalai Lama also saw the creation of a patronage relationship between the emerging Qing (Manchu) Dynasty in China and religious rulers.

The Fifth Dalai Lama established three medical schools during his reign. The site selected for the third school was on a mountain named "Iron Mountain," or Chagpori, a prominent peak outside Lhasa. A decree established that each of the large monasteries near Lhasa, as well as those in surrounding districts, would receive a physician of its own from the Mentsikhang—literally, "house of medicine and astrology."

During the reign of the Thirteenth Dalai Lama (1895–1933), a gifted physician and scholar, Kyenrab Norbu (1882–1962), founded the Lhasa Mentsi Khang in 1928. This new college provided a place for one student from each provincial monastery to study, as well as offering opportunities for private students.

Shangri-La

Tibet's geographic and political isolation through the late nineteenth and early twentieth centuries made its traditions an object of curiosity and speculation in the West. This fascination manifested itself, for example, in the story of a hidden paradise, Shangri-La, described in the best-selling novel of the 1930s, *Lost Horizon*, by James Hilton (1933). Tibet became the purview of military adventurers, arcane scholars, and intrepid explorers, like the fictional Indiana Jones of the late twentieth century. Ultimately, Tibet's isolation would work to its disadvantage.

Paradise lost

In the invasion of Tibet by China in 1959, by the People's Republic of China, much of the material culture of Tibet was lost or destroyed, and traditional Tibetan culture began to be actively suppressed. Tibetans in exile have made substantial efforts to protect and nurture the cultural and spiritual traditions developed in their society for more than a millennium, yet Tibetan medicine is a tradition in exile and in flux—consequences of the "liberation" of Tibet on its medicine cannot be undone.

Outside of what is now known as the Tibetan Autonomous Region (TAR) of the People's Republic of China (PRC), most efforts to preserve the tradition are coordinated by the Tibetan Government in Exile and particularly by the Mentsi Khang (the Tibetan Medical and Astrological Institute), which was established on March 23, 1961, in Dharamsala, Himachal Pradesh, India. Dr. Yeshi Dhonden served as the first head of the medical section. The preservation of medical teachings and the sponsorship of medical training by Tibetans living outside of the PRC are undertaken by a number of teachers, physicians, and centers throughout India and other parts of the world.

Within the PRC, Tibetan medicine falls under the purview of the State Ethnic Affairs Commission and the State Administration for Traditional Chinese Medicine (SATCM), which in recent years have made an effort to establish several colleges of Tibetan medicine and hospitals that provide training and practice resources for Tibetan medicine.

Although the development of Tibetan medicine outside Tibet faces a lack of economic and political resources, the tradition within the TAR faces the challenges posed by the profound religious components of the medical system, which are fundamental to understanding aspects of Tibetan medicine. The practice of Buddhism in Tibet is viewed as a potential focal point for political resistance, and because many of the major religious figures of Tibet are in exile, the integration of religious perspectives into what is intended to be a state-sponsored approach to indigenous medicine poses profound problems.

The (vanishing) world of Tibetan medicine

The world of Tibetan medicine is composed of the five elements, which provide the basis for understanding the body. The metaphorical structure of the three roots of Tibetan medicine— theory, diagnosis, and treatment—is used to organize the concepts and practices.

At the basis of theory, the universe and the body are each results of the interplay of the five elements. Wind, fire, water, earth, and space are the constituents of the universe and all that is contained within it (Table 7.1).

Each of the first four of the elements—earth, fire, air, water—is represented by a set of qualities to describe the associated organs, functions, tastes, and seasons. As examples, earth gives rise to the olfactory organs, fire permits the process of digestion, wind (or air) presents rough and light tastes, and water dominates the winter season. The fifth element—space—provides the area in which the other four elements interact, and comprises, as well as the openings and cavities within structures formed from the other four elements.

The five elements are energies, or dynamic forces, which deal more with their inherent energetical function rather than any actual state. One finds all five elements in any substance. They are, however, present in different proportions. for example, when it is said that a phenomenon is composed of the fire element, this means that the fire element predominates, and that the phenomenon manifests fire qualities most distinctly.

Thus, substance and structures may be gross, subtle, or very subtle, and these distinctions pertain to the ease with which structures and substances may be experienced on the basis of sensory perception or meditative insight.

In the mythical tradition that informs the Tibetan worldview, the earth is said to be supported by a subterranean ocean of water. Underneath this is a great fire, which is fanned and kindled by a region of wind below it. This image depicts the five elements in the matrix of space. In this universe, the change of climate with the seasons is caused by the activity of the wind, which stirs up the fire, heating the ocean waters and producing spring and summer.

The interaction of the four elements in the matrix provided by the fifth, space, is a powerful metaphor for the experience of "emptiness" (sunyata), which can be equated with the absorption of all phenomena into an egoless, spacelike awareness of unconditioned selflessness. The experience of emptiness is a prerequisite for the gradual attainment of enlightenment in the Buddhist tradition. When you take a handful of earth and put it in water it dissolves; if you heat up water with fire, it vaporizes; if you blow excessive wind on the fire, the fire goes out; and when the wind is still, then there is nothing.

In Vajrayana (Tantric) Buddhist practice, the energies/elements are personified as five Wisdom Buddhas, who are heads of "families" that share their characteristics. These Buddhas, often depicted in instructive and devotional art, are used as a system for encountering and working skillfully with the energies in meditation, and more widely in whatever guise

Table 7.1 The Five Elements

Wisdom Buddha family	Element	Type of wisdom	Enlightened qualities	Deluded qualities
Vairochana	Space	Integrative	Peace; the capacity to abide; simplicity	Avoidance; denial; withdrawal
Aksobhya	Water	Mirrorlike	Seeing things as they are; knowing and explaining	Controlling; fear of chaos; anger and hatred
Ratnasambhava	Earth	Equanimity	Accommodating; sharing common humanity	Self-absorption; neediness; greed and possessiveness
Amitabha	Fire	Discriminating	Intimacy; caring and compassion	Malignity; overly competitive and manipulative
Amogasiddhi	Wind	Accomplishing	Doing what needs to be done; inspiration and spontaneity	Need for power; jealousy and envy

they are met. They are applied in the practice of medicine, and in understanding personalities and relationships—when constituted as a system of individual personality types, revealed in the description of the characteristics of the deluded mind and the enlightened mind of each family, as presented as part of Table 7.1.

Anatomy in Tibetan medicine: channels and organs

Tibetan anatomical concepts are similar to those described in the texts of Ayurveda and Chinese medicine, but differ in some particulars. For example, the enumeration and description of the skeletal system may be inadequate from the perspective of systematic, bioscience-based anatomy. However, it is critical to recognize that the organization of these structures guides surgery, and still is the basis for locating structures for the more aggressive methods of therapy in Tibetan medicine: venesection, cautery, and acupuncture.

The concept of channels (Tibetan: *rtsa*) is essential to the theory and practice of Tibetan medicine. Channels are differentiated in a variety of ways, and the term rtsa itself takes its meaning from context and qualifiers. It can have the sense of a distinguishable anatomical structure, such as vein, artery, nerve, or lymph vessel. A "white" channel (*rtsa.dkar*), for example, is typically nervous tissue. A channel can be "subtle" pathway, which conveys subtle winds (vital energy), and is accessed in meditation. In diagnostics, *rtsa* can convey the sense of a pulse, and the palpated artery itself is a channel through which wind and blood flow. Channels are extensively described and mapped. A clear conception of the channels permits an understanding of the movement of vital substances in the body, and the ability to locate channels permits the palpation and treatment of specific vessels.

The organs in Tibetan medicine are divided into the solid five organs, or viscera (*don.lnga*), and the six hollow organs, or bowels (*snod.drug*). These organs share certain similarities with the viscera and bowels (Chinese: *zang fu*) of Chinese medicine, especially in being simultaneously real tissue structures and related to both physiological function and the surface of the body.

Concepts and human conception

In the Buddhist view of conception, the body of a human is formed when the red seed of the mother, the white seed of the father, and the very subtle mind and wind combine during sexual intercourse. From a Buddhist view, the very subtle mind is the aspect of consciousness that bears, from life to life, the effects of previous actions. At death, it absorbs the less subtle aspects of mind that are most familiar in ordinary consciousness.

The various stages of fetal development are dealt with extensively in Tibetan medical texts. The five elements, under the influence of karma, reflect the actions committed in past lives that bring about the new human body.

The father's sperm forms the bones, brain and spinal cord, and the mother's blood forms the flesh, blood, solid organs and hollow organs. The (five) sense consciousnesses arise from one's own mind (i.e., the mind of the being who enters the mother's womb). The flesh, bones, organ of smelling, and odors are formed from the earth element. The blood, organ of taste, tastes, and the moisture (in the body) arise from the water element. The warmth, clear coloration, the organ of sight, and form arise from the fire element. The breath, organ of touch, and physical sensations are formed from the wind element. The cavities in the body, the organ of hearing, and sounds are formed from the space element. According to Dr. Yeshe Dhonden, everyone living on this planet has taken birth in dependence upon the five elements. We rely upon them for the necessities of life, and likewise, all medicines are composed of the five elements.

Even death takes on a pattern derived from the interaction of the five elements. Death begins with the sequential dissolution of the winds associated with the four elements—earth, water, fire, and wind. "Earth" refers to the hard factors of the body such as bone, and the dissolution of the wind associated with it means that wind is no longer capable of serving as a mount or basis for consciousness. As a consequence of its dissolution, the capacity of the wind associated with "water"—the fluid factors in the body—to act as a mount for consciousness become more manifest. This pattern of dissolution continues through all the elements. As death occurs, the five elements are experienced sequentially as their subtle aspects are absorbed before the departure of consciousness from the body.

From their relation to the universe, conception, fetal development, the essential components of the body, death, and medicine, the five elements are fundamental to all phenomena and life processes.

The three roots of the tree

Tibetan medicine is seen metaphorically and structurally as a tree, with three roots that functionally delineate the system. The first root is the theoretical understanding of the healthy body in contrast to the diseased body. The second root is the diagnostic system, involving observation, palpation, and questioning of the patient. The third root comprises treatment modalities, including, diet, medicines, and behavioral and spiritual interventions.

The first root, the first trunk, and the three humors

Translated as the "Root of the Actual Situation of the Body," the first root has two trunks. The first trunk describes the components of a body in a balanced state, uncharacterized by disease. However, the very nature of the vital substances of the body implies a tendency toward imbalance and disturbance. Thus the first branch of the first trunk presents the three faults, or the "humors"—wind (Sanskrit: *vayu*), bile (*pitta*), and phlegm (*kapha*) (compare Table 6.1).The Tibetan term for the faults is *nyes.pa*; its Sanskrit counterpart is *dosha*. The term is often translated as "humor," because of the recognizable similarities between the four humors of Greco-Roman medicine (black bile, yellow bile, blood, and phlegm). However, the Tibetan and Sanskrit terms *nyes.pa* and *dosha* denote something that is "faulty," or whose character is inherently "defective." In this sense, "fault" more clearly reveals the meaning, because these vital substances—wind, bile, and phlegm—are faulty by their very nature. They are prone to increase, decrease, and disturb, which results in disease. For this reason, the branch that describes them is called the "disorder branch."

The three humors are formed from the five elements in the following manner: phlegm from earth and water, bile from fire, and wind from wind. Space provides an environment for the activities and interactions of the elements and furnishes the openings and cavities of the body, but it is not a component of the humors.

Phlegm has the combined qualities of earth and water and is supported and increased by the presence of these elements. If we imagine the mud that results from the combination of water and earth, we have a good idea of the characteristics of phlegm. It is moist, unctuous, and cold. In balance, phlegm contains nutrients, lubricates joints, and facilitates the smooth functioning of the body. Where present in excess, phlegm produces heaviness, dullness and sogginess. The amount of phlegm that the body contains is three double handfuls.

Bile has a hot nature and is responsible for heating and transformation within the body. Bile gives the body color and supports vision. When disturbed or present in excess, bile can cause pathological heat and disturbance in many organs. The amount of bile in the body is that which would fill the scrotum.

Wind is a mobile substance responsible for all aspects of movement in the body, from walking and respiration to the transport of vital substances and constituents. Wind is characterized in some contexts as essentially neutral and in others as cold. In terms of wind's role as a vehicle of the other humors, it can be said to be neutral. Alone, wind is said to have a cold nature. The amount of wind in the body is just the amount contained in an inflated urinary bladder.

Where wind is regarded as a cold humor, some consider blood as a fourth humor. Blood is also regarded as an important constituent of the body and is generally considered to be hot. This schema that uses four substances indicates that Persian and Arab traditions based on the four humors of Greco-Roman medicine (Unani) have been incorporated into the Tibetan system.

In the description of the healthy body, the three humors are shown to carry out actions that correspond to their qualities.

Phlegm produces a moist, soft substance, which is transformed by the heat of bile, and the resultant products are moved through the body by the wind. Each stage in the process of digestion is shown to be accompanied by tastes that are associated with the currently dominant humor. The metaphorical tree of Tibetan medicine represents a healthy body by describing the first trunk as bearing two flowers and three fruits. These are the flowers of health and longevity and the fruits of spiritual practice, wealth, and happiness. Health and longevity are considered the basis for all fundamental worldly and spiritual attainments.

The first root, the second trunk

The second trunk of the first root is the body characterized by disease. It has nine branches that cause illness to be produced. Concepts of specific diseases include an understanding of contagious diseases, and of diseases caused by very small, difficult-to-see organisms.

The first branch, substantive causes, has three leaves: desire, anger, and ignorance. These causes are the emotional afflictions familiar to students of Buddhism. Thus, the causes of imbalance—the humors or faults—lie in the past actions of body, speech, and mind, in what are called "distant" causes. Desire is the distant cause of wind, anger the distant cause of bile, and ignorance the distant cause of phlegm. "Distant" means a span of many lifetimes and rebirths, connected by the cause-and-effect relationships (*karma*) that, from a Buddhist point of view, condition our existences. From this perspective, it is understood that the actions taken in past lives produce the results that we experience in the present. At the root of these distant causes lies the fundamental ignorance of the nature of reality. Thus, according to the Explanatory Tantra the sole cause of all disease is said to be ignorance due to lack of understanding of the meaning of "emptiness" or selflessness.

The second branch, co-emergent conditions, has four leaves: time or season; harmful influences such as spirits, inauspicious days, and unfortunate planetary aspects; unbalanced diet; and inappropriate behavior. Generally, the co-emergent conditions act directly to imbalance the faults, by furnishing conditions whose qualities or elemental character interact with them by similarity (Ergil 1983, 2006), exacerbating the tendency of a fault to imbalance, or by opposition, diminishing the actions of the humors or faults to which they are opposed.

Seasons and climates promote or suppress humors. In some cases the humors can be disturbed in one season, while the disorders emerge in another. An example is the disturbance of phlegm that occurs in the winter, only to emerge in the spring as the newly warm season reveals its character.

The status of spirits is problematic in a modern age. The Buddhist worldview is capable of simultaneously accepting a spirit as a reality and as the manifestation of a disturbed mind. Some authors have expended great effort to establish the spirit world of Tibetan medicine as form of psychiatry, it is important to note that the malign influence of spirits was a part of the Tibetan world. On this basis, the diagnosis of spirit-caused disease has been a relevant response to disease. Within the diagnostic tradition there are specific methods for determining the role of spirits in diseases.

Diet, for example, is fundamental both to the cause and the cure of disease. Inappropriate foods are foods that are consumed to excess, in the wrong combination, at the wrong time, or by the wrong constitution. If an individual partakes of sweet foods to excess, the phlegm becomes unbalanced and leads to decrease in digestive heat. Since earth and water elements constitute phlegm, they are constituents of foods having a sweet taste. Digestive heat is produced through the fire element and is a healthy manifestation of the digestive bile. Fire is quenched and cooled by water, so an excess of the water element in the diet will damage the digestive fire.

Past behaviors associated with the "three poisons" of desire, anger, and ignorance are thought to be the cause of current disorders. Current behaviors also may lead to an imbalance of the humors and create karmic consequences in future lives. From the point of view of Buddhist medicine, avoiding anger can reduce the likelihood of bile disorder both in this life and in future lives. Other mental and emotional extremes can disturb the humors as well. For example, grief and intense mental activity can disturb wind. Other behaviors that disturb the humors are those that stress or alter the customary body rhythms. To suppress or restrain a natural function, such as suppressing a sneeze or an urge to urinate, can trigger wind disorders. Strenuous work under the wrong conditions can produce the heat of a bile disorder.

Further branches

The detail of all nine branches of the characteristics of the body in disease is comprehensive. It is enough for our purposes to touch in on some further areas of significance.

Disease is said to first affect the skin. Subsequently, the muscle tissue, channels, and then the bones are affected. After that, the disease passes into the five viscera and then the six bowels.

The general locations of the humoral disorders in the body are those associated with their characteristics and with the areas typically governed by the actions of the humor in health. Thus, wind disorders are often associated with the hips and waist. This pertains to the role of wind in activities such as movement, excretion, and reproduction. Bile disorders are associated with the middle of the body, because its seat is the liver. Phlegm is considered to have its seat in the brain, so its disorders frequently affect the upper body. Distinguishing the periods during which a fault will predominate permits the physician to anticipate occasions when specific diseases will flourish. This practice also permits the activities and diet of a patient to be guided according to seasonal and environmental influences and the nature of the disease.

The sixth branch, the time of arising, has nine leaves, which are classified in three divisions according to (1) age, (2) seasons and times, and (3) region. This branch is particularly instructive, as we can see clearly how a relationship continues to be created between the qualities of an event and the nature of a given fault. There are three relationships drawn in the division of age: phlegm arises in youth; bile predominates in middle age; and wind characterizes elderly people. There are three relationships in the division of region: wind places are cold and breezy; bile places are dry and tormented by heat; and phlegm places are very moist and oily. There are three relationships in the division of seasons and times: wind illness arises in the summer time, evening and dawn; bile imbalances occur in the autumn, midday, and midnight; phlegm produces disease in the winter, at dusk, and in the morning.

The seventh branch deals with the result of disease (death) in all its manifestations. The eighth branch discusses the possible transformation of the disorder through the suppression of one humor while another becomes unbalanced. The ninth branch has only two leaves, dividing the humors and blood into hot and cold.

The second root: recognition of signs

The root of the recognition of signs (diagnosis) has three trunks: (1) the trunk of the science of observation, (2) the trunk of the science of examination by feeling, and (3) the trunk of communication skills, questioning and hearing. Observation involves examination of the tongue and the urine, as well as observing the bearing and facial coloration of the patient. Feeling the pulse allows the practitioner to assess whether a disease has its origins in wind, bile, phlegm, or a combination of these and to understand which organs are affected. Questioning of the patient is used to evaluate prior behavior and current symptoms to determine the nature of the illness. All three of these diagnostic modes organize bodily information into signs that represent the state of the body to the physician and allow him or her to understand the nature of the patient's disease. These signs reveal the characteristics of disease, which then reveal the affected humors.

The third root

Treatment, the third root of Tibetan medicine, is to a great extent simply the ways of reversing the disease state as theorized and diagnosed in the first two roots. We have spent enough time with the theory for such a discussion to be more tedious than enlightening—particularly as the possibilities for westerners to experience such treatments continue to wane.

Pure Buddhist medicine

Tibetan medicine is not available on a general basis in the West, and has been threatened in its home of origin due to the circumstances ongoing between China and Tibet. It is, nonetheless, among the world family of healing traditions, perhaps emblematic of what can be called Middle Asian medicine, and the pure form of what can be called "Buddhist medicine," while representing, to considerable extent, the intersection of medical knowledge from India, the Middle East, Ancient Greece and Rome, and China in a dynamic form.

While Tibetan medicine was disappearing, and the ability for it to be experienced by westerners was limited, it survives in essence and (as shown on the cover illustration) may be said to represent the "central" Middle Asian tradition; literally and figuratively, central in terms of time, place, and eclectic incorporation of all the wisdom on offer by this largest (by geography and population) region of the globe. As we have shown throughout this book, concepts of the vital healing of mind, enery, consciousness and spirit form a unity among these medicines. The Appendix to this book provides a practical guide to accessing and experiencing the type of healing consonant with these Middle Asian insights and traditions; through the widely available, preserved and reincarnated therapies of Ayurveda, the mother of Tibetan medicine, which in its geneology also claims the many fathers identified in this chapter.

Chapter 8

The Lights of Healing

Unani Medicine and the Greco-Arabic *Tibb* System

The contributions of Arab and Muslim physicians to medicine are widely perceived to have originated in their translations of ancient Greco-Roman medical texts, and their subsequent elaboration and evolution of the material presented in those texts. In fact, the word *Unani*, used as the name of the system of medicine they developed, is an Arabic adjective meaning "Greek." These scholar-practitioners worked to create methodical approaches to disease etiology, prognosis, and diagnosis; to systematize medical practice; to build organized hospitals and clinics; to expand the repertoires of drugs and catalogs of surgical instruments; and to establish professional ethical codes. Unani medicine (or *Tibb*, its Arabic common name) thus represents a vital link, fertile ground, and prerequisite to modern medicine that developed later in the West during the decline of the Arab-Muslim Empire.

The comprehensive and encyclopedic books transcribed by Unani physicians led to the widespread practice and teaching of this system in Europe from the time of the Renaissance, as well as in other parts of the world for centuries. Nonetheless, the present-day Unani medical system is restricted to South

Asia, where it has survived alongside Ayurveda and Siddha. The limited recognition of Unani by the West is probably due to the interest in developing and exporting the more pervasive Ayurvedic system. (It should be noted that Unani Tibb is recognized by the World Health Organization (WHO 2002) as an alternative system of medicine.)

There is often a suggestion that Unani is so close as to be almost similar to Ayurveda; however, these two systems also have fundamental differences. While the practical aspects of Unani medicine present similarities, the theoretical as well as some philosophical aspects are different from Ayurveda regarding the seat and sources of vital energy. Although Unani has a more discreet concept of the individual spirit (*nafs*) and its role in health and healing, the concept and role of spirit in Ayurveda is more collective and ultimately more diffuse, more like a collective consciousness.

There is also a general perception that Unani is specifically a Greco-Muslim and not generally a Greco-Arabic medical system. However, Unani physicians were not all Muslims, but also included Jews (Rabbi Moses ben Maimon, 1134–1204, known as Maimonides), Christians (Hunayn *Ibn Ishaq*, 808–873, known as Johannitus), and Persians, all of whom wrote and practiced in Arabic, because it was the language of the political elite and the sciences in the Golden Age of the Arab-Muslim civilization that spanned Spain to Central Asia for over 600 years. Arabic was also, of course, the language of Islam, the religion that eulogized knowledge and tolerance. Among traditional medical systems, Unani represents a complete system of practice with highly developed physical diagnosis.

Looking back at the light

Looking back, it has been said that Islamic medicine reflected the light of the ancient Greek sun, and when its day had ended, it then shone like a moon, reflecting that light, and illuminating the darkest night of the European Middle Ages. And by this light, the dawn of a new day in Europe—the Renaissance—arose.

Unani practices can be traced back nearly three thousand years to their Egyptian and Mesopotamian roots, where the Greek historian Herodotus and the physician Hippocrates (c. 460–370 BCE) traveled, and where the Roman physician Galen (c. 129–199 CE) studied and practiced medicine. The walls of Egyptian temples and burial sites, and Egyptian papyri (such as the Edwin Smith papyrus), as well as some Sumerian clay tablets from Mesopotamia, provide fragmentary records. In addition, the works of Hippocrates, Dioscorides and Galen provide a more thorough record of ancient medical knowledge, primarily through subsequent translations by Arab and Muslim scholars during the Middle Ages. These works were expanded by Arab and Muslim physicians such as Rhazes and Avicenna, who added from their own experience and pertinent observation. (Rhazes is Abū Bakr Muhammad ibn Zakariyā Rāzī (Arabic: أبوبكرمحمد بن زكريا الرازي; Latin: Rhazes or Rasis), chemist, physician, philosopher and scholar. Rāzī was born in Rayy, Iran, in the year 865 (251 AH) and died there in 925 (313 AH); Avicenna is Abū 'Alī al-Ḥusayn ibn 'Abd Allāh ibn Sīnā (Arabic: أبوعلي الحسين بن عبداللهبن أبي سينا); born c. 980 near Bukhara, Khorasan, died 1037 in Hamedan, also known as Ibn Seena.) They corrected misconceptions and recorded their own discoveries, such as alcohol extraction of medicinal plants and distillation of rose oil, the distinctions between infectious diseases such as small pox and measles, and explanations of meningitis and pleurisy. Rhazes focused on infectious diseases, while Avicenna identified over 750 drugs, and emphasized preventive medicine, exercise, diet, and mental health.

Rhazes and Avicenna authored the texts *Al-Hawi* and *Al-Qanoon* respectively. The former is considered the largest ancient medical encyclopedia, and the latter became the standard medical textbook throughout most of Europe for hundreds of years, until the development of chemistry and modern medicine. Unani medicine was the catalyst and vehicle for revival, modernization, and systematization of ancient Egypto-Greco-Roman medicine that laid foundations for modern medicine.

An allopathic Western medical system in Europe evolved from knowledge embodied in the Unani tradition, during the eighteenth and nineteenth centuries. Unani medicine also ultimately provided a source for other natural, holistic, and alternative practices like homeopathy, naturopathy, and chiropractic in Europe and the United States.

Like other of these holistic medical traditions, Unani medicine also included psychological evaluation as an intrinsic part of all patient examination (an early approach to mind-body medicine). In addition to physical signs, the Unani physician also used both mental and emotional characteristics to determine the temperament of the patient.

Though technically rudimentary, the Unani methods of diagnosis represent an excellent understanding of biological systems and states of health and disease. These traditional methods of patient examination offer cost-effective, real-time evaluation of patient status where the caregiver does not have to rely on calibrated machines and delayed test results to treat an illness.

Culture and history: a familiar and unfamiliar background

The regions of the Eastern Mediterranean, Near East, and Middle East were a cradle of human civilization. Following a nomadic subsistence, here humans first formed permanent settlements and irrigation agriculture, growing early crops and domesticating animals. Here, alphabetical letters were invented and used. Here, sciences and religions were developed and spread. Here, likewise, is the home of the ancient system of Greco-Arabic medicine known as Unani. When studying Unani medical traditions, one can trace the continuity of medical knowledge from ancient Egypt, to Greece and Turkey, to Syria and Iraq, on to Pakistan and India, where it resides today

In the pre-Christian era, ancient Greece and Rome appear in reality to have been very different culturally than what was constructed in Europe later as the "Classical Period." Greece and Rome were not so much continuous parts of European civilization, as an integral part of the contiguous African, Middle Eastern, and Arabic regions.

In the pre-Islamic era, Persian influences constantly intersected, sometimes violently, with ancient Greece. Following the establishment of Islam, first in Arabia, then spreading to North Africa to the east and India, and ultimately Indonesia, to the west, Middle Eastern influences were a nearly permanent situation in Greece from the time of the Arabs to the Turks of the Ottoman Empire in the early twentieth century, with the modern fault lines still being felt on the island Cyprus and elsewhere.

Culturally, ethnically, and historically, Greece was part of an Eastern Mediterranean and Middle Eastern continuum. This part of the world, in the aftermath of the break-up of the Ottoman Empire after World War I, is where successive European powers have ventured at their peril: the British Empire, the Russian Empire and then USSR, and currently the United States. While the Hashemite Arabs in their struggle for independence were enlisted as part of the larger theatre of conflict in World War I, the Arabian Peninsula itself passed to the Kingdom of Saud, and the British placed their Hashemite allies on the thrones of Jordan (to this day) and Iraq (where later the Bath Rebellion of the 1970s placed Sadam Hussein, for a time, in charge)—a story now well known to American and British readers.

Harmony in nature and cosmos

All traditional medical systems harmonize the health of the individual with the universal elements of nature and the cosmos—with vital energy. They all seek a balance between opposing, but complementary, elements. Unani, in ways similar to Chinese medicine and Ayurveda, adheres to a holistic and balanced approach to health maintenance, diagnosis of illness, and restoration of health. It assists the natural recuperative power of the body; recognizes all factors that contribute to human health status; and avoids harming sound parts of the body when pursuing treatment options for a disease.

Unani's theoretical basis encompasses the theory of naturals (*tabie'iat*) a unifying explanation of the shared natural building elements of the universe and humans, which classifies the normal constituents and functions of a healthy individual. Unani practice is based on the theory of causes (*mousabibat*) that identifies the elements underlying illness, and on the theory of signs (*'alamat*) that identifies diagnostic symptoms.

The naturals (*tabie'iat*)

Avicenna defined Unani medicine as a branch of knowledge based on physical laws, the naturals (*tabie'iat*), and not on dogma or superstition. There are seven main sets of naturals that form the essential constituents and the working principles of the body: elements or phases (*arkan*); temperaments (*mizaj*); humors (*akhlat*); organs (*a'dha'*); faculties (*quwa*); functions (*af,* افـا); spirits (*arwah*).

"Elements" or phases (arkan, ان كـار*)*

The elements are also known in Arabic as the basics, or origins (*ousoul*). The four elements are earth, water, air, and fire. A fifth energetic element, the aether, is considered the source of the other four, but is not used in Unani medicine. The ancient philosophers of the Levant attempted to formulate a unifying theory that explains all natural phenomena—just as in contemporary physics. Because in their time they lacked the tools for molecular and atomic investigations, they used symbolism to hypothesize, predict, and substitute for the unknown, and referred to objects by their characteristics rather than their constitutions. For example, the elements also represent all physical phases of the matter: solid, liquid, gaseous, and energy. They considered these physical phases as the elements that form the ingredients of everything in the universe, including humans. Their usage in medicine confers their characteristics to the body, its organs, and its energies.

Avicenna described the earth element as "a simple motionless heavy object that occupies the center in a group of elements. It helps life forms attain cohesiveness, shape, and stability" (anticipating the Newtonian concept of gravity). He also described the physical relationships among the elements, "the water element engulfs the earth, and the two are surrounded by air." He placed the fire element as the connector between the other three elements, and attributed to fire the bringing of the earth and water from their elemental states into compounds by reducing their inertia. His characterization of the fire element is similar to a modern description of free energy. Furthermore, he pointed out that the air and fire are constituents of the life energies. From this work, we can see that Avicenna was more broadly a natural scientist than what we would consider a medical scientist, or a physician, to be today.

Each element is associated with fixed qualitative characteristics (nature/temperament) called the "elemental powers." These are hot, cold, wet or moist, and dry. Each element possesses two such powers: earth is cold and dry, water is cold and wet/moist, air is hot and wet/moist, and fire is hot and dry. Additionally, earth and water are associated with heaviness, and fire and air with lightness. Heavy elements are thought of as strong, negative, passive, and female, while light elements considered weak, positive, active, heavenly, and male.

The four elements are dynamic, interacting and resulting in continuous change within the human body; the change is either cyclical or directional. The food and water cycles are examples of cyclical change, whereas an abnormal growth of a tumor represents a directional change. Because the elements have to exist in equilibrium to maintain health, any change in the elements is monitored to assess the health status of each part of the body. This monitoring is accomplished through the temperaments (*mizaj*).

Temperaments (mizaj, مزاج)

The literal meaning of *mizaj* is the quality or qualities of a mixture. Its classic use means that temperament is a product of the opposite physical qualities of the four elements (hot, cold, wet, and dry). It is the sum quality of the body, or any of its organs, due to the actions and reactions of the elements. Its definition can encompass the metabolic, behavioral, and psychological profiles of the individual, and can also be considered a physical state or phenotype. Individuals acquire a temperament phenotype during their life, due to their genetic predispositions, environmental effects, and lifestyle choices. It is important to understand the theory of the temperaments, because certain conditions are associated with a particular temperament, meaning that normal signs of one temperament are abnormal in others. Further, the temperamental phenotype determines the suitability of a treatment and suggests the dose of medication.

There are four basic elemental temperaments: hot, cold, wet, and dry. However, because these four can also occur in combinations, the total number of temperaments is nine—eight inequables and one equable (balanced). The eight inequables result from the unequal presence of the opposite qualities, these encompass four temperaments of single qualities—hot, cold, wet, and dry—and four composite temperaments: hot and dry, hot and wet, cold and dry, and cold and wet. Because the elements are constantly interacting, the normal balanced state for each temperament has a range. Humans have a body temperament range that differs from animals; age groups and geographic races have their own ranges; and healthy ranges are different from ranges of illness. Additionally, each organ has its own temperament with ranges of heat and cold, wetness and dryness. For example, the hottest are breath, blood, liver, flesh, and muscles; the coldest are phlegm humor, hair, bones, cartilage, and ligaments; the wettest are phlegm humor, blood, oil, fat, and brain; and the driest are hair, bone, cartilage, ligaments, and tendons.

Humors (akhlat)

The term humor is derived from the Greek chymos ($\chi\upsilon\mu\acute{o}\varsigma$, juice or sap). However, humoral theory is ancient and cannot be attributed to a single person or tradition. Most of the humoral descriptions reference Hippocrates, whose writing on the subject survived. The four humors are present in the bloodstream in different quantities, and are considered the essential components of the body that occupy the vascular system. Later, Avicenna concurred with Hippocrates and added the tissue fluids (inter- and intracellular) as the secondary humors.

Balanced humors are considered the source of health, and restoring the humoral balance is the basis of Unani treatment to restore the health of sick individuals. Unani adheres to the humoral theory with four humors: blood (*dam*), phlegm (*balgham*), yellow bile (*safra'*), and black bile (سوداء). Ancient Greek medicine had used only three humors, blood, phlegm and bile, until Thales of Miletus (c. 640–546 BCE), who had been educated in ancient Egypt, aligned Greek traditions with Egyptian medical concepts by adding the fourth humor, the black bile. Similar to the elements, each humor has two natures: blood is hot and humid, phlegm is cold and humid, yellow bile is hot and dry, and black bile is cold and dry. Thus, there is a correspondence between the natures of the human body and the natures of objects in the physical world.

The temperament of the individual results from the proportions of the four humors. There are four basic types of temperaments named for the predominant humor: sanguine (blood humor predominates, *damawi*), phlegmatic (phlegm humor predominates, *balghami*), bilious or choleric (yellow bile humor predominates, *safrawi*), melancholic (black bile humor predominates, *saudawi*). Various combinations also commonly occur, as with the Ayurvedic kapha, pitta and vata,

In their healthy state, each individual has a unique equilibrium humors that maintained by vital forces or powers called *quwa*)—the metabolic strength and functions of organs. Emphasis is placed on diet and digestion for the restoration of humoral balance and health, and on the restorative power of quwa, fortified by prescribed medications.

Organs (a'dha')

Based on structure, organs are classified into two types: simple and compound. The simple organs are homogenous in structure such as bones, nerves, tendons, veins, and arteries; while the compound ones are heterogeneous and composed of several other organs—the head, for instance, is a compound organ.

Unani medicine assigns primary importance to four organs: heart, brain, liver, and gonads. The heart is the essential distributor of the two vital energies (*pneuma* and *ignis*); the brain controls the mental faculties, senses, and movement; the liver carries out the nutritive and cleansing processes; and the gonads give masculine and feminine characteristics and temperaments, and form the reproductive elements.

Faculties (quwa, ىوق-ـلـا): psycho-physical drives

A faculty is a capability or a potential. The faculties constitute the biological systems of organs and their physiological processes. There are three major faculties: the vital or animalistic (*hayawaniyyah*, ـح-ـي-ـناوـيـه), the psychic (*nafsaniyyah*, نـفـساـنـيـه), and the natural or physical (*tab'iyyah*, طـبـعـيـه). Each of these faculties carries out its functions under its corresponding spirit and have identical locations as their spirits. Vital faculties are the source of the motive energy (the Life Force that is referred to as *Thymos* (θυμος) by Classical Greeks); they are either the active type that is involuntary like heart beat, or acted upon (voluntary) such as emotions of anger, happiness, and contempt. Psychic faculties represent the conscious and unconscious mind and perform three functions: underlying behavior, stimulating voluntary movement, and generating sensation.

The natural faculties have a hierarchical relationship since they fall into those that serve other faculties and those that are served by others. For example, the nutritive faculty is served by four others: the attractive, the retentive, the digestive, and the expulsive. These four serving faculties serve the nutritive faculty by attracting, retaining, digesting, and expelling; and the nutritive faculty serves the growth faculty, which with the forming faculty, serve the generative faculty.

Functions (af'al, ـلـا-ـعـف أ)

The functions complement the faculties, where each faculty has its specific functions emanating from specific organ. Avicenna classifies functions into single (such as digestion) and compound (such as eating which requires the desire for the food, taste, and swallowing).

Spirits (arwah): life energies

These spirits differ from the theological and mystical ones, and are purely physical "energies of life." Their uses in Unani medicine signify the deriving forces or energies that help the faculties connect and carry out their functions. Arab/Muslim and Greek physicians divided these energies into two types: *pneuma* (breath, *nafas*), analogous to the oxygen needed for cellular aerobic respiration, and *ignis* (fire, *har*, حـ-حرار) thermal energy produced by physiologic respiration needed for digestion and metabolism. *Pneuma* is "pure, warm, light, and mobile air," while ignis is responsible for providing the heat or energy needed to carry out metabolic processes.

Lungs take *pneuma* from air, mix it with blood, and send it to the heart where it gets distributed throughout the body organs, and attains various functions by these organs. Unani physicians attributed functions to *pneuma*, not organ differentiation, and divided *pneuma* into three forms within the human body on the basis of source and function: the natural, the psychic, and the vital. The vital or animalistic spirit (Greek: *pneuma zoticon*; Arabic: *hayawaniyya*, حيواويه) stems from the heart, and functions to preserve life by preparing suitable conditions for the other two spirits. The psychic spirit (*pneuma psychicon*, *nafsaniyyah*) originates in the brain, and stimulates sensation and perception through the cognitive faculty, and triggers movement through the motivation faculty. The natural spirit (*pneuma physicon*, *tab'iyyah*) derives from the liver, and is associated with the nutritional and reproductive processes performed by the natural faculties.

Ignis as the fire or energy produced in the presence of air, *pneuma*; *ignis* does not exist without *pneuma*. It is the energy that drives all metabolic processes within the body, and is responsible for the body's innate heat emanated during these metabolic processes. Like *pneuma*, *ignis* occurs within the same major organs and assumes similar names.

There is a striking similarity between this ancient explanation of the body's energies and our current knowledge of respiration physiology. In modern scientific interpretation, the *pneuma* and *ignis* are equivalent to oxygen intake and its important functioning role as the electron acceptor in the cellular mitochondria. The chemical energy of respiration generated free heat as adenosine triphosphate (ATP) and provides the cells with its energetic currency.

The causes of disease (*mousabibat/alasbab*, باسباب/التبببسم)

For humans to maintain good health, six essential factors have to be present: (1) fresh clean air, (2) food and drink, (3) movement and rest, (4) sleep and wakefulness, (5) eating and excreting, and (6) a healthy mental state. A long-term disruption of these essentials results in illness. Illness affects the functions of the vital, psychic, or natural faculties due to an imbalance or obstruction of a temperament (dystemperament) or a combination of functions and temperaments. Unani physicians state that the body has three health conditions: (1) healthy (i.e., disease-free), (2) ill or diseased, and (3) a continuum between the two: in situations when the disease is still in its asymptomatic phase (which may manifest as a functional complaint or disorder prior to the detection of symptoms) or when recuperating from a symptomatic phase. The third state may manifest in three forms: (1) disease affects only one organ while the rest of the body remains healthy, (2) healthy state is not optimal as in aging individuals, and (3) health and illness alternate in a temporal fashion as in individuals with hot temperament who are ill in the summer but well during the winter, or vice versa.

Dystemperament is either local or systemic, and involves one or more of the four basic qualities: hot, cold, wet, or dry. The effect is usually added from an outside and often unexpected source. On the other hand, humoral illness involves metabolic disorder, which results in the imbalances and/or corruptions of one or more of the four humors. The disorder is either quantitative (excess or deficiency), qualitative, or both simultaneously. Most humoral disorders originate internally due to metabolic errors that result in excess (anabolism), such as high triglycerides, or wasting (catabolism), such as degenerative diseases or cancer.

Unani medicine (like Ayurveda) attributes the origins of most illnesses to the corruption of the *pepsis*: the digestive and metabolic processes (generation and distribution of humors). According to Alkindi "the stomach is the house of all illness" (Alkindi is Abū Yūsuf Ya'qūb ibn Isḥāq al-Kindī (Arabic: وبأ يوسف يعقوب إبن إسحاق الكندي), c. 801–873 CE, known in the West as Alkindus). He advised not to eat when angry, and not to bathe on full stomach. The conditions under which digestion occur are as important as the diets that are consumed.

On a daily basis, the individual encounters potentially pathogenic stresses; however, most of these fail to cause illness. They only cause disease when the individual's resistance and adaptive responses have been weakened or compromised and the virulence of the pathogen overwhelms the host's defenses, or the pathogen is able to establish itself through a weakness in the host systems.

Signs of imbalance ('*alamat*, تامال-ع)

Evaluation of an individual's health takes into consideration innate traits (*lawazem*, مزاول), such as age, gender, race, skin complexion, and geographic adaptations. Traits attributed to long-term multigenerational adaptation to living in a particular geographic area should not be confused with signs of temperamental imbalance. For example, people from warm equatorial regions of the world have hot temperament, as well as dark complexion, eyes, and hair, while those from temperate zones have cold temperament, as well as light skin, eyes, and hair. Thus, the cold temperament of Northerners is not an indication of a phlegmatic state.

Age also dictates different assessments depending on its phase. Four phases of life are recognized: youth (from birth till 28 years of age), adulthood (ends at 40), maturity (ends at 60), and old age (ends at death). Because bodily functions vary in their efficiency for each phase, each is also associated with its own innate temperament: youth is hot and wet; adulthood is hot and dry; maturity is cold and dry; and elderliness is cold and strangely wet. Therefore, *age temperament* should be considered before considering an *organ's temperament*; the prescribed diet and herbal treatments should be suitable for the age group. There are also some traits that develop in relation to age progression that should not be confused as symptoms of illness. For example, hair thinning and a desire for naps are associated with the phases of maturity and older age and are not indicative of an imbalance. These life changes should be accepted as normal with aging, rather than requiring medical intervention. Thus, the popular modern notion of "anti-aging" has no place in Unani thought or practice.

Avicenna described a set of traits to be examined by the *Hakim* (م-ي-ك-ح, Unani physician) to determine temperamental status: the quality of skin texture and complexion (should be slightly moist, warm, smooth, elastic, and between white and red); balance of muscle and fat; hair characteristics (should be full, thick, between straight and curly, balanced growth in location and length); organ configuration; reaction time of faculties; dreams; and balance of sleep and wakefulness.

Also, the *Hakim* looks for signs of humoral excesses where all the humors are over abundant, or deficient, or one is in excess at the expense of another. Other signs are characteristics of stool and urine, stomach growling, mouth odor, nail shape, cheek color, involuntary movements (e.g., cough, spasm, shivering), congestion and blockage, gas formation and blockage; and tumors. Special attention is given to fevers, tongue color and texture, pain, pulse, and the eyes.

Imbalance of temperaments (dystemperament)

The first diagnostic feature is a dystemperament of the ailing organ or system. There are four main dystemperaments: hot (hotter than usual, but not moister or drier); cold (colder than usual, not moister or drier); dry (drier than usual, not hotter or colder); moist (more moist than usual, not hotter or colder). These states are dynamic—constantly changing and interacting.

Dystemperament can affect an organ, tissue, or a system, and may include any of the humors or a combination of them. Dystemperaments are determined by the signs of the body or an organ; and they are either qualitative (indicative of a disease) or material and spatial (indicative of the location). The dystemperament is qualitative if it is not bound within an organ directly (as with a fever), and is material if it is within an organ and causing changes there (e.g., a cold liver will produce pale urine and light stool).

After gathering information about the patient, the *Hakim* tries to identify the form of humoral imbalance.

Imbalance of humors

Humoral disorders emanate from corruption of the pepsis (digestion and metabolism within the body), which fall under the natural faculty. Nowadays industrial chemical pollutants can cause humoral disorders if they enter and persist in the body. When the humors are undersupplied and underperforming, the metabolic process is weak, which leads to problems in the functions of the systems and organs. Underperforming humors tend to generate more phlegm and less blood. When the humors are oversupplied, metabolic processes are overactive, leading to an unbalanced oversupply of metabolites, which is toxic to the system. This toxic accumulation loads the body with black and yellow biles.

Although humoral disorders are metabolic in nature, the humors may get dystemperamented like any other part or organ of the body. Coldness, dryness, and wetness slow the humors down, while heat puts them in overdrive.

The symptoms and diseases usually associated with each of the humors are shown in Table 8.1.

The *Hakim*

Hakims rely on their senses, knowledge, reasoning, and experience to gather all signs of imbalance and reach a diagnosis. In addition to the medical history of the patient, the *Hakim*, through observation and physical exam, gathers the physical and mental signs of imbalance. The physical examination encompasses the tongue, nails, pulse, urine, feces, and the presence of pain and fever.

The *Hakim* determines the patient's humoral temperament from three sets of characters: (1) appearance (complexion, build, touch, hair), (2) physiological (movement, diet preferences, seasonal preferences, sleep, pulse), and (3) emotions (calm, angry, nervous, etc.). The patients' humoral imbalance manifests itself in their mental status, behavior, and mannerism. States of these traits can be attributed to one of the four humors:

Table 8.1 Signs of humoral imbalance

Blood	Angina, bleeding disorders, canker sores, constant erection and convulsion of penis, coughing, cracked nails, delirium, diphtheria, enlarged tongue, excessive menstrual flow, gout, headache, heart disease, hemorrhoids, high blood pressure, lethargy, loose teeth, migraine, nose bleeding, nose itching, pleurisy, poor vision, slackness of uvula, swelling of liver, swollen palate, swollen testicles, tooth spaces, trembling lips, uremia, weak limbs
Phlegm	Acne, arthritis, asthma, atonic dyspepsia, backache, bad breath, bad taste in mouth, baldness, boils, canker sores, chronic bronchitis, colic, conjunctivitis, constipation, constriction of throat, continuous trembling, convulsion of stomach, convulsions, corrupt appetite, cough, dandruff, dandruff of eyelids, deficient appetite, dilation of pupils, diphtheria, dull feeling in teeth, enlarged tongue, erectile dysfunction, forgetfulness, foul odor from nose, gripe, headache, heart feels as if being pulled downward, insomnia, itching of anus, joint ache, lethargy, madness, melancholy, muscular tension, obstruction of liver, paralysis, pimples, pleurisy, respiratory allergies, retention of urine, ringing in ears, scabs, sebaceous cysts, severe perspiration, severe thirst, shedding eyelashes, sour mother's milk, styes, swelling of bladder, swelling of lips, swelling of liver, swelling of lymph nodes, swelling of spleen, swelling of testicles, swelling of uvula, swelling of womb, swollen eyelids, swollen palate, trembling limbs, ulcers of gums, ulcers of kidneys, upset stomach, vomiting, weak limbs, weak nail growth, whiteness of lips
Yellow bile	Anal ulcer, biliousness and biliary congestion, boils on eyelid, burning urination, canker sores, cough, delirium, discolored teeth, dull teeth, excessive appetite, excessive menstrual flow, feeling of "smoke" in chest, gall stones, gastric and duodenal ulcers, gastritis, gripe, hard eyelids, headache, heart attack, hemorrhoids, hyperacidity and acid reflux, insomnia, jaundice, migraine, nose itching, photophobia, pleurisy, rheumatoid arthritis, swelling of liver, swelling of testicles, tendonitis, vomiting, yellowed nails
Black bile	Abnormal growths and hard tumors, arthritis, cancer, canker sores, clots and embolisms, colic, constipation, delirium, diphtheria, excessive appetite, excessive libido, flatulence, gripe, hallucinations, headache, heartburn, insomnia, insufficient mother's milk, intestinal obstruction, irritable bowel, neuralgia, seizures and convulsions, skin cancer, stiffness, swelling of bladder, swelling of liver, swelling of spleen, swelling of stomach, swelling of womb, thickened nails, varicose veins, vomiting

- A sanguine personality is usually balanced, stylish, refined, passionate, positive, genial, inquisitive, playful, sensual, and indulgent.

- A phlegmatic is calm, good natured, trusting, sluggish, inactive, sentimental, sensitive, loving, subjective, self-absorbed, and steady.

- A choleric is forceful, energetic, flamboyant, expressive, dramatic, bold, fidgety, short-tempered, angry, and argumentative.

- A melancholic is quiet, cool, aloof, detached, objective, withdrawn, cautious, prudent, frugal, stoic, stiff, inflexible, moody, and grumpy.

The *Hakim* is usually on the lookout for behavioral and personality signs that may provide a clue to the patient's illness.

Diagnostic tools

Traditional medical systems use many of the same techniques to spot the signs of deviation from the normal range in order to determine the malfunctioning organ(s). The conditions of pulse, tongue, urine, and feces are used as diagnostic tools.

Pulse (nabd, ضبن)

The heart is the distributor of pneuma to the rest of the body and directly determines the vitality of the system (the production of free energy and chemical energy). The Unani system of pulse diagnosis was developed by Avicenna. He had studied all the available pulse information of his time, and then integrated all in his synthesis. Galen and Avicenna understood the challenging nature of pulse diagnosis as evident in their writings. Practicing *Hakims* admit that it is the hardest part of *Tibb* to master.

A pulse is composed of two movements corresponding to the heart beat (systole and diastole), with rests following each of the movements. The pulse is felt at the radial artery near the wrist, where it is closer to the skin surface and easily accessible.

To examine the pulse, the *Hakim* places the middle finger on the radial artery, directly between the carpus and the prominence of the radius bone, with the other two adjoining fingers next to it in their natural positions and the index finger proximal to the heart. It is recommended that the pulse of a female be examined on the right hand, and the left hand for a male, with the palm turned upward for both.

Pulse evaluation—ten characteristics

Avicenna listed ten characteristics of pulse evaluation. The first seven determine whether the pulse of an individual is regular, these are as follows:

The first seven

1. dimensions of expansion (length, width, and depth)

2. strength as a force felt against finger (strong, moderate, weak)

3. speed (fast, moderate, slow)

4. compressibility (soft, hard, and in between)

5. turgor: tension of the artery between pulses—fullness (full, empty, and in between)

6. temperature of the pulse (hot, cold, and in between)

7. duration of diastole (short, long, and in between).

The next three

8. regularity (regular in all preceding characteristics), or irregular

9. order and disorder in irregularity

10. rhythm, specific to the individual and usually measured as the ratio between the two movements and the two rests.

Seven compound pulse types
Further, Avicenna classified the irregular pulse into seven compound pulse types:

1. gazelle

2. wavy

3. wormy/cordlike/twisting

4. antlike

5. sawlike

6. mouse-tail

7. snake-tongue, needle-like/flickering.

Considering elemental temperament, a hot temperament, if healthy, is associated with "great pulse," the best type of pulse, while a cold temperament has a weaker pulse. A wet temperament produces a wavy and wide pulse, and a dry one is associated with tightness and stiffness and produces spasmodic and shaky pulse. Further, considering humoral temperment, a sanguine temperament (hot and moist) has a moderate to slightly rapid pulse that is moderately soft and relaxed; phlegmatic (cold and wet) has a deep, slow, and soft pulse; melancholic (cold and dry) has a slow to weak, tense or constricted, thin, and well-defined pulse; and choleric (hot and dry) has a strong, rapid, and well-defined pulse.

Tongue (lisan, لسان)

There are two areas of interest in the tongue: the body and the coat. The tongue body reflects the temperament and blood supply within the body in general, while the tongue coat reveals the health of digestive and metabolic processes, and humoral imbalances.

The tongue body texture is indicative of systemic or chronic conditions that are severe. Its texture could range from dry or rough, cracked, raw, rumpled, to wet and glossy. These conditions may indicate lack of body moisture, nervousness, advanced sickness, inefficient digestion, and excess moisture respectively.

The tongue coat's color, size, and texture are all taken into consideration for diagnosis. The coat reflects the health state of digestion, digestive tract, and metabolism, and its surface location reflects the affected part of the system (pancreas, intestine, stomach, liver, etc.). An absent to a thin coat denotes a good digestive and metabolic health, while an increase in thickness reflects poor digestion, and thickness is proportional to the accumulation of metabolic toxins in the body. Coat color indicates the nature of the buildup (phlegmatic, choleric, etc.) and its texture reflects moisture content.

Urine (boul, لبول)

The urine provides a window on the metabolic status of the individual. Avicenna stated that the urine is indicative of the health of the liver, urinary tracts, and blood vessels. He stressed several specifics for urine collection in order to derive accurate assessment. For example, it should be the first collection of the day before the individual eats any food. The individual should have had no food the night before that might color the urine, have had no intercourse, and should have been resting for a while before urination. *Hakims* assess the urine within the first hour of its collection by evaluating its quantity, color, foaminess, texture, clarity, and sediment. Avicenna eliminated touching and tasting the urine as part of the evaluation.

Urine may have a few colors depending on the individual's state of health, ingested food, water intake, or drugs. Its color can assume the following shades and hues: yellow, red, green, black, and white. For example, shades of yellow may range from straw yellow, lemon yellow, blond yellow, orange yellow, fiery yellow (saturated yellow), to saffron yellow with a tinge of red. The first two indicate a normal heat temperament, while the rest indicate increased heat, or may be generated by extreme exercise, pain, hunger, or thirst.

Feces/stool (bouraz, بوراز)

Feces, also called alvine discharge, have characteristics that are indicative of the individual's *pepsis* and health. Normal feces are yellowish in color, cohesive with uniform softness similar in its consistency to unfiltered honey; it comes out easily without burning sensation, air sounds, or foam. Its quantity is compared to the ingested food amount; a reduced amount is thought to be due to retention in the tract, while an increased amount points out the presence of humors. Wet feces (as in diarrhea) indicate weak digestion, weak absorption, or blockage, while hard feces (as in dehydration) may point out excessive urination, ingestion of dry food, prolonged retention, or fiery heat within the system. The color of the feces specifies the affecting humor; for example, a dark or black color is a sign of a maturation of a melancholic disease (if one can exclude excessive heat, colored diet, or a drink that emits black bile).

Pain (waja', ألم)

Pain is considered an unnatural condition for the human body, and should be transitory in nature. It is usually caused by a dystemperament or an injury—loss of continuity. Pain weakens the organs and halts their functions; it warms initially but later cools down and saps energy. Removal of the cause will eliminate the pain, which is the preferred method of treatment (e.g., applying a poultice of linseed (*Linum usitatissimum*) or dill (*Anethum graveolens*), or by applying wet sedatives (alcohols), or cold anesthetics (all narcotics)).

Pains and their causes

Avicenna listed fifteen types of pains and their causes:

1. itching (*hakak*, ح-كاك), caused by a humor that is bitter or salty

2. rough (*khashin*, خ-ش-ن), caused by rough humor

3. stabbing (*nakhes*, س-خ-ان), caused by a humor extending the muscle membrane and separating it

4. flattening/extended (*moumaded*, د-دمم), caused by a humor or gas pulling the nerve or muscle from two opposite ends

5. pressing (*daghet*, ط-غ-اض), caused by a substance engulfing the organ and pressing on it

6. splitting (*moufasekh*, خ-س-فم), caused by a substance seeping out of the muscle or its membrane and separating the two

7. breaking (*moukaser*, ر-س-كم), caused by substance, gas, or coldness in between the bone and its membrane

8. softening (*rakhou*, رخ-و), caused by extending only the muscle without the tendon

9. boring (*thaqeb*, ب-ق-اث), caused by the trapping of gas or substance between the tissues of a hard organ such as the colon

10. piercing (*masalee*, م-س-لي), caused by the boring of a hard organ by a gas or substance

11. dull (*khader*, ر د-خ), caused by a cold temperament, or obstruction of blood supply

12. throbbing (*dharabani*, ض رب-ا-ن-ي), caused by hot inflammation next to an organ

13. heavy (*thaqeel*, ث-ق-ي-ل), a sense of heaviness in an insensitive organ such as lung, kidney, or spleen due to inflammation or tumor, or when the tumor disables the pain sensation, such as cancer in the mouth of the stomach

14. tiring (*a'ya'i*, ا-ع-ي-ئ-ي), could be due to fatigue, or by an extending humor, a gas, or ulcerative humor

15. biting/incisive (*lathe'*, ع-ذال), caused by a sour humor.

Fever (*homa* [s], *homiat* [p], ح-م-ى، ح-م-ي-ات)

In the fourth volume of his Al-Qanoon, Avicenna wrote a detailed study on fever types, symptoms, causes, and treatments. Fever is an unnatural heat "centered within the heart and spirits" (i.e., involving *pneuma* and *ignis* energies), and carried throughout the body by blood and the vascular system. It is a disquieting sign of corruption and imbalance that requires attention. On the basis of origin, there are two main classes of fevers: (1) fevers associated with infections (*waba'yah*, و-ب-ا-ئ-ي-ه), and (2) transient fevers associated with warming effects, foul humor, hyperplasia, and blockage. On the basis of their causes and locations, the second class has three types of fevers: (1) ephemeral fevers (*homa youm*, ح-م-ى ي-وم), (2) humoral fevers and putrefactive fevers (*homa khalt/'ofounah*, ح-م-ى ع-ف-ون-ه خ-لط), and (3) organ fevers and hectic fevers (*homa daq*, ح-م-ى د ق).

Avicenna attributed the infection and its associated fever to the contamination of air and water with "malevolent soil objects" that are taken into the body. These "objects" corrupt the body's "spirit" and produce unnatural heat that spreads throughout the body. However, he ascribed the infection's success to the presence of corrupt humors, which permits the infection to take place.

Ephemeral fevers

All ephemeral fevers are caused by external warming effects: sun's heat, exhaustion, hot food and medications, sports, and emotional tension. These fevers usually last one day (hence the name *youm*, which means a day in Arabic), and rarely up to three days. However, a fever lasting beyond three days signifies that it has spread to an organ or a humor, and therefore could turn into a putrefactive or hectic type.

Putrefactive fevers

Putrefactive fevers are caused by corruption of the humors. They arise in the body due to the ingestion of contaminated food (and the effects of its byproducts), high-moisture fruits, incomplete digestion, and lack of oxygen (possibly, improper breathing). Putrefaction may affect the whole body, or an organ, or a humor. Because putrefactive fevers are associated with humors, they are classified according to the affected humor: (1) *alghibb* fever (ح-مى الـغـ-ب), an alternating fever, day on/day off, caused by the putrefaction of yellow bile humor; (2) *mutbiqah* fever (ح-مى مطـبـقـه), consistent and caused by the putrefaction of blood humor; (3) *na'bbah* fever (ح-مى نـائـبـه), caused by the putrefaction of phlegm humor; (4) *alroub'* fever (ح-مى الـربـع), which cycles one day on and two days off, and is caused by the putrefaction of black bile humor.

Organ fevers

Organ fever (or hectic fever) may follow after the other fever types mentioned above. It is considered difficult to diagnose but easy to treat at its incipience, easy to diagnose at its end but difficult to treat, and untreatable if the patient withers. Organ fever affects the moisture at three stages: at the first stage it reduces moisture in the vessels; at the second stage it reduces moisture between the tissues and produces wilting (*thoubool*, الذبول), and at the third stage, decomposing (*moufatit*, متفتم), it reduces moisture within the tissues.

Unani health maintenance, prevention, and treatment of disease

Unani medicine emphasizes healthy practices of exercise and diet for health maintenance and prevention of sickness. Avicenna divided medicine into theoretical and practical, and further subdivided the practical into two sections: (1) management of healthy bodies, he also called it the "science of health preservation," and (2) management of sick bodies.

Health is maintained by the proper internal balance of heat and moisture that allows the innate heat to be generated and participate in the proper functioning of the body. The body uses the food to generate its needed energy and as building blocks to maintain structural integrity of the body.

Exercise (riyadhah, الرياضة)

Avicenna placed exercise at the forefront as the most effective means for health maintenance. He claimed that regular exercise prevents dregs from accumulating in the body. Additionally, exercise increases the innate heat, lightens the body, strengthens muscles and tendons, as well as prepares the organs to take in nutrients, reduces their stiffness, and prevents their weakness.

The *Al-Qanoon* section on exercise is extensive, and lists a large number of general physical exercises, such as running, archery, speed walking, jumping, horseback riding, wrestling, rowing, and many others, as well as specific organ exercises designed for eye and ear, for example. It also instructs on the time of exercise and on preparing for it, and goes on to describe the types of fatigue and other conditions that result from exercise and the methods to treat them. This section also encompasses the use of massage and steam bath.

Diet for health and healing (alghitha', ءاذـغـلا)

Heath is maintained by food that is balanced in quality and quantity. However, excretion does not get rid of all unutilized food material; there are residues that remain in the body that keep accumulating over time. These dregs have a bad effect on the body: their byproducts will harm the body; their accumulation in larger quantity leads to dystemperament; and their overload will produce the diseases of excesses (أمـرارض ءالتـمالا). Accumulation of dregs in an organ produces tissue enlargement, and the spread throughout the tissues corrupts the *ignis*. Expulsion of dregs is usually facilitated by poisonous drugs or by detoxification. When dealing with humoral imbalance, a ripening of the humoral substances is carried out first, usually with laxatives, followed by purging.

The process of detoxification is carried out to rid the body of accumulated dregs (toxins, superfluous matter). Over a period of a few days, the individual deviates from their regular daily diet to take in food and drink that will induce detoxification. This process culminates in a "healing crisis" or catharsis of elimination where the elimination may take place as diarrhea, nosebleed, perspiration, urination, or vomiting. There are many recipes for detoxification by food ingestion or administration of enemas; however, it should not be carried out more than once a year.

Recognizing that humans have different needs at their various life stages, Avicenna described the types of diets that should be followed for infants, pregnant and breast-feeding women, adults, and elderly individuals. He also described and treated the various conditions that may arise from those diets due to excesses or imbalances for each age group.

Therapeutic diet in Unani medicine is used to restore balance by means of providing the proper food that suits the temperament of the individual and their digestive system. Such diet entails the elimination of unsuitable food, low-quality or contaminated food, excesses of one type, and unhealthful mixtures; reduction in the number of meals; and the introduction of foods that stimulate digestion, breathing, circulation, and innate heat, such as spices, vegetables, and oils.

Medicinal substances (dawa', ءاودـلا)

Treating with medications (botanical, zoological, and metallic substances) is the second choice for treatment after diet. Unani herbal usage is extensive and well documented in many old texts that are still in current use. These treatments cover almost all known diseases. Unani *Hakims* use single and compound formulas as well as internal and external applications.

There are three rules to treating with medications: the first is to know the temperament of the medication (hot, cold, moist, dry); the second, to determine the quantity to be given to the patient and its effect (warming/cooling, drying/wetting); and the third, to determine the most effective time of its administration. Selection of the medication follows the diagnosis of illness. As a rule, the medication is opposite in its temperament to that of the disease. However, the characteristics of the diseased organ determine the quantity of the medication. These include its temperament, architecture, position, and strength. For example, the quantity of the medication should correspond to the amount of deviation from the normal temperament. Additional factors are also considered for calculating the quantity, such as patient's strength, gender, and age, as well as time of the year (season), and geographic location.

Food and medications are ranked according to their power to affect the human body into eight classes: four degrees for hot food and medications and four degrees for cold ones. Unani formularies always give the power degree; for example, a medication is usually followed by "hot in the second degree" or "cold in the third degree."

Herbal treatments can be applied in a number of methods such as capsules, conserve, decoction, essence, fomentation, infusion, ointment, oxymel, plaster, poultice, salve, suppository, syrup, and tincture. Use of aromatic oil and alcohol extracts is featured prominently in Unani treatments. Avicenna invented steam distillation of rose oil. Alcohol extraction and preservation of active ingredients of botanicals was discovered earlier by Arab chemists and put to use by *Hakims*.

Manual therapy ('elaj, ج-ال-ع)

Bleeding is used for blood humor, purged through a procedure of bloodletting from a vein called *venesection* (*fassd*, د-ص-ف-ل-ا). Two main conditions require venesection: (1) excess of blood, and (2) low quality of blood. However, venesection should be carried out at the early signs of some diseases, such as varicose vein, gout, joints pain, high blood pressure, epilepsy, and melancholy. Using leeches (*al'alaq*, ق-ل-ع-ل-ا) is another method for bloodletting through placing leeches on the skin of the patient. They attach to the skin by their oral suckers, and remain there until they get full and fall off to digest. This method is still in use today in both East and West.

Cauterization

Cauterization (*alkaiy*, ي-ك-ل-ا) is the application of heated metal or a corrosive directly to the skin surface. It is considered a treatment of last resort, due to its harsh effects. One of its main purposes is to prevent disease from spreading to healthy parts of the body. However, it is also applied to infected areas, unhealthy flesh, and to weak parts—for strengthening.

Cupping

Cupping (*hijameh*, م-ا-ج-ح-ل-ا) is an external application of vacuum suction to the skin in order to draw humors to the surface, away from an organ or area. It is used to treat inflammation and for detoxification. The type of disease determines the location of cupping. For example, cupping on the heels is beneficial in amenorrhea, gout, and varicose veins, while on the sides of the neck it affects the head's organs. Cupping is not advised for people over 60 years of age.

Enema

Enema (*houknaeh*, ه-ن-ق-ح) is an effective method for emptying the intestines (especially after vomiting), reducing kidney and bladder pain and enlargement, and detoxifying of upper organs. However, a harsh enema may weaken the liver and produce fever.

Massage

Massage (*tadleek*, كـيـل دتـلـل) and bathing (*istihmam*, أسـتـحـم-ا م) are ancient traditions in the old world that can be considered one integral activity. It takes place in a warm bathhouse (*hammam*, م ا-حـم) that is usually built on a fresh water source. It starts with a vigorous cleansing rub with a soapy loofa (*leefeh*, لـيـفـه), usually a dried fruit of *Luffa* plant or a linen mitt. After a good rinse, an oil massage is applied with hands, fingers, and palms, with various pressures depending on the treatment goals.

Not all of these therapeutic modalities would be selected as offerings in a CAM or integrative medicine clinical program nowadays. Unani shares much with the other systems of medicine we have reviewed so far. It also provides a bridge between East and West, and between ancient modern medicines, shining a light on the paths medicine has taken to bring us to the present. Unani medicine is not just a recapitalization of ancient Greco-Roman healing. Rather, it added its own creative dimension, in conceptualizing the human body in continuity with the physical world, as well as in anticipating in its own way some of the thinking about the nature of reality found in modern physics.

Chapter 9

Rapid Healing

Sufism in the Middle East

The history of Sufism dates back about 1500 years to the time of Muhammad and the birth of Islam. Muhammad was born in Mecca and lived from 570 to 632 CE, in what is now Saudi Arabia. He was an orphan by age six, and was taken in by his uncle Abu Talib. At age 25, he worked as a merchant for a widow, Khadija, transporting goods to Syria. Khadija was 15 years older than Muhammad, but was so impressed with his character, and perhaps his youthful vigor, that she later proposed marriage to him. They were married for about a quarter of a century until her death, during which time he never took other wives, even though polygamy was common practice.

Muhammad would frequently retire for meditation to a cave, later known as "Hira," on top of a mountain north of Mecca called "Nur," or light. At age 40 in the year 610, while meditating in that cave, it is said he received the first of a series of divine revelations through the angel Gabriel. These revelations continued over 23 years through this "unlettered" prophet, and were memorized and written down by his followers, and became the Qur'an, or the holy text of Islam.

The Qur'an consists of 114 chapters. It has not been modified since it was written down. Thus, it is the same text today as was revealed during Muhammad's lifetime. Tradition holds that the Qur'an is divinely protected from being corrupted (verse 15:9). The Qur'an is also notable for its internal consistency and its external agreement with historical and archaeological evidence, as well as for providing new information and scientific findings that did not come to light until the nineteenth and twentieth centuries. For example, it vividly describes human fetal development well before the dawn of scientific knowledge of embryology (Qur'anic verses 22:5, 23:12–14, and 40:67). Muhammad is not worshiped or seen as divine, but rather is credited with the revelation of a literary masterpiece, along with the founding of a major religion and a new world power, although the latter has made for complex international relations.

The terms "Islam" and "Muslim" were never meant to represent an exclusive religion, or an elusive practice, but rather to present the universal concept of peace through "surrendering oneself to the will of Allah" (the Arabic word for the God). Therefore, a Muslim is one who surrenders his or her whole self to the one God. In fact, all living creatures, including animals and insects, are seen as natural Muslims, following divine design by their instinctual behaviors. However, it is only humans who can choose either to surrender to the will of Allah or to rebel and follow their own selfish desires. This struggle between surrender and rebellion represents the history of the evolution of human moral consciousness or the process of spiritual Jihad as described later in this chapter, with Allah sending prophets to lead people back to the creator. Also, Islam presents itself as a religion of peace, as expressed in the letters that form the word "Islam" from "Salam," which means "peace." In addition, one of the "beautiful names" of Allah as described in the Qur'an is "Al-Salam." Further, the greeting of the believers is peace, or "Asalamualaikum." Finally, believers are ordered to spread "Salam." Although to present-day westerners it may appear that a few followers may not have kept to this sacred principle of spreading peace in Islam.

Peoples of the Qur'an

The Qur'an teaches that Allah sent the same basic religion and revelation to humans, without holding one of the earlier religions above the later ones, including Judaism, Christianity, and Islam. These teachings are revealed in the Old Testament, New Testament, and Qur'an. This universal religion was revealed to the first human, Adam, and all the earlier prophets: Noah, Abraham, Ishmael, Isaac, Jacob, Joseph, Moses, Aaron, David, Solomon, Zachariah, John, and Jesus. As stated in the Qur'an:

> The same religion has He established for you as that which He enjoined on Noah—that which We have sent by inspiration to thee—and that which We enjoined on Abraham, Moses, and Jesus; Namely, that ye should remain steadfast in Religion, and make no divisions therein. (42:13)

Contrary to popular belief, and the proclaimed views of modern Islamic fundamentalists, Islam is not anti-Judaism or anti-Christian but commands that all Muslims respect and revere all the previous messengers, books, and messages revealed to them. Because Jews and Christians received earlier revelations from Allah, they are referred to as "People or family of the Book" in the Qur'an. Thus the Qur'an holds that Allah's universal message has come to people across the ages through appointed messengers as a type of "progressive revelation" (2:106). The form of this message may change according to the needs of the people and their circumstances, but it is the same basic message of surrender to the will of Allah. Thus, the true Islamic view is acceptance of these other religions as noted in the Qur'an: "The Messenger believeth in what hath been revealed to him from his Lord, as do the men of faith. Each one (of them) believeth in Allah, His angels, His books, and His Messengers" (2:285).

Islam also sees people as equals, only distinguished by their righteousness:

> O mankind! We created you from a single (pair) of a male and a female, and made you into nations and tribes, that ye may know each other (Not that ye may despise each other).

> Verily the most honoured of you in the sight of Allah is (he
> who is) the most righteous of you. (49:13)

In addition to the believing in prior messengers and scriptures,
the central belief of Islam is in the Oneness of God (Allah). Not
only is there just one God, but also God (Allah) is in control of
everything in the universe, regardless of whether we humans
judge outcomes in the world as positive or negative. Islam also
accepts the existence of angels and the Day of Judgment and
that Muhammad is the last prophet and the Qur'an is the last of
Allah's holy books.

The way of the Sufi

Sufism is the mystical spiritual tradition within Islam, which
directs humans toward a "nearness" to the God (Allah) so that
they can become agents for Allah. As noted in the introduction
of the Qur'an (Abdullah Yusuf Ali edition):

> For the fulfillment of this great trust man was further given
> a Will, so that his acts should reflect Allah's universal will
> and Law, and his mind, freely choosing, should experience
> the sublime joy of being in harmony with the Infinite, and
> with the great drama of the world around him, and with his
> own spiritual growth.
>
> But, created though he was in the best of moulds,
> man fell from Unity when his Will was warped, and he
> chose the crooked path of Discord. And sorrow and pain,
> selfishness and degradation, ignorance and hatred, despair
> and unbelief poisoned his life, and he saw shapes of evil
> in the physical, moral, and spiritual world, and in himself.
> (C:1)

Thus the spiritual tradition of Sufism represents the direct path
back to Allah or, as noted in the Qur'an's "Opening" Surah 1:6,
"the straight way."

The Sufi musician Hazrat Inayat Khan (1983) provides the
following description of spiritual development:

> The word "spiritual" does not apply to goodness or to
> wonder-working, the power of producing miracles, or to

great intellectual power. The whole of life in all its aspects is one single music; and the real spiritual attainment is to tune oneself to the harmony of this perfect music. (Khan 1983)

The foundation of Sufism is based on belief in the mystical aspects of the spirituality of the Prophet. During his lifetime, pious individuals from different nations learned under his guidance the Spiritual Laws of Islam, because these laws led toward direct experience of the Divine or nearness to Allah.

The Shaikh

The spiritual leader of a Sufi school is known as a Shaikh. The spiritual knowledge of the Shaikh can be traced back to Muhammad, who later converted his cousin and son-in-law "Ali bin abi Talib." Ali is considered a spiritual heir to the Prophet and the one who inherited his spiritual knowledge and power. Thus, all Sufi Masters are his students, directly or indirectly; this is the origin of the title "Shaikh of the Shaikhs." Through a line of succession, each Shaikh would initiate a successor based on revelations from Allah, maintaining a direct spiritual link or attachment with Muhammad to the present spiritual leader. This chain down to the present Master of a Sufi school is known as the silsila. At present, there are more than 150 orders or schools of Sufism.

A Shaikh is a mediator or guide in Sufism to help the student draw near to Allah, battle their lower self (jihad), and help channel the spiritual power from Allah to perform paranormal phenomena (discussed under the metapsychology of Sufism). As noted by the teachings:

The mediator is essential. Ask your Lord for a physician who can treat the diseases of your hearts, a healer who can heal you, a guide who can guide you and take you by the hand. Draw near to those whom He has brought near to him, His elite, the ushers of His nearness, the keepers of His door. You have consented to serving your lower selves and pursuing your passions and natural inclinations. You work hard to satisfy and satiate your lower selves in this world, although this is something that you will never achieve. You keep to this state hour after hour, day after day, month after month and year after year, until you find that death has suddenly come to you and you cannot release yourselves from its grip. (Chishti 1991)

If Allah did not reveal someone with the attributes that qualify the person to be a Shaikh, the Shaikh would not name a successor, and the silsila of that particular tariqa (way) would discontinue. In such a case, for example, the dervishes would have to join another tariqa after the departure of their Shaikh to maintain the spiritual link necessary for the attainment.

The unifying factor and ultimate aim of the Sufi way is the attainment of "nearness" to Allah by means of following a chain of masters who have already attained nearness to Allah and by following the path. This process of drawing near also is related to purifying one's lower self through personal internal struggle, or jihad. The process of drawing near to Allah may include the acquisition of paranormal powers, such as rapid wound healing and paranormal knowledge, including Qur'anic knowledge. One of the great Sufi masters, Shaikh "Abd al-Qadir al-Gaylani," used to describe what the dervish would obtain as being "something that no eye has ever seen, no ear has ever heard, and has never occurred to any human heart" (2:74). In Sufi terms, the attainment to Allah means the transformation into light by becoming absorbed or extinct in the Light (i.e., Allah). Allah describes Himself in the Holy Qur'an as being "nur" (light): "Allah is the Light of the heavens and the earth" (24:35). The nearer the dervish draws to Allah, the more Allah attributes he acquires. When the dervish achieves the ultimate goal of total "extinction" (Arabic: *fana*) in Allah, he will lose his own will and become an instrument in the hands of Allah, thus experiencing the ultimate submission of one's will to Allah. With this nearness to Allah, one can reach the high stage of being an agent (viceregent) for Allah, with spiritual guidance, vision, and power to help transform peole and the world. The broad implication for society is having an umma, or community, united by following the will of Allah versus the traditional tribal, blood, and kinship allegiances with accompanying blood feuds that were so prevalent during the original times of Muhammad and again today—and pretty much at all times in between (Armstrong 1993).

Sufism is not associated with terrorism or fundamentalism. The Sufi spiritual viewpoint may not be generally accepted by some traditional Muslims; it has even been met with hostility from other Muslim schools of thought. Of course, traditional Muslims accept that righteous living in this life will lead them to Allah and in the next life, but Sufi, as with other mystical traditions, believe that one can gain direct experience of Allah in this life by following the spiritual path.

The straight path to the divine

An integral part of Sufism is the notion of a "path" or "way" toward Allah through self-understanding, certain practices, and discipline. Thus, Sufism is the straight path, or one of the shortest paths, to God. Many great spiritual traditions use the concept of a path or way toward the experience of the divine. For example, Buddhism is known as a path toward Nirvana or enlightenment (Chapter 7). In the Bible, Psalm 25:4 states, "Show me thy ways, O Lord; teach me thy paths." Continuing with verses 9–10, "The meek will he guide in judgment: and the meek will he teach his way. All the paths of the Lord are mercy and truth unto such as keep his covenant and his testimonies." In the New Testament, Jesus said, "I am the way, the truth, and the life; no man cometh unto the Father, but by me" (John 14:6). Similarly, in the beginning chapter of the Holy Qur'an, Al Fatihah ("The Opening") 1:6–7, Allah teaches the people how to pray to Him in these verses: "Show us the straight way, The way of those on whom Thou hast bestowed Thy Grace, Those whose portion is not wrath, and who go not astray."

Straight path, straight posture

The idea of a spiritual path has a corollary within the Western philosophical concept of "means" versus an "end." As John Dewey (1922) noted when discussing means and end concerning an activity:

> The distinction of means and end arise in surveying the course of a proposed line of action, a connected series in time. The "end" is the last act thought of; the means are the acts to be performed prior to it in time. To reach an end we must take our mind off from it and attend to the act that is next to be performed. We must make that the end. (Dewey 1922)

Dewey's concept of means and end were greatly influenced by the mind-body movement therapy work of F. Matthias Alexander (1910). Alexander observed that many postural problems people encountered were caused by unconscious movements to gain some end, such as sitting or standing, without much thought as to the means, way, or path of accomplishing this goal. Alexander taught individuals to focus on the "means whereby" of doing a simple act such as the process of moving from sitting to standing versus focusing on the end results or "end gaining," as he termed it. The process of attending to the "means" or "way" resulted in increased conscious guidance and control of the self. As Alexander noted:

> This triumph is not to be won in sleep, in trance, in submission, in paralysis, or in anaesthesia, but in a clear, open-eyed, reasoning, deliberate consciousness and apprehension of the wonderful potentialities possessed by mankind, the transcendent inheritance of a conscious mind. (Alexander 1910)

From this perspective, following a path or way or attending to a means may be associated with increased awareness or consciousness, or perhaps even a higher consciousness comparable to the increased consciousness or awareness found in one's body movements following instructions with the Alexander method (Alexander 1910) or the Alexander technique of bodywork today.

The five pillars of Islam and Sufi Healing

As a spiritual tradition within Islam, Sufism follows the five pillars of Islam: the statement of belief or Shahada ("There is no God, but The God [Allah] and Muhammad is the messenger of Allah"), prayer, fasting, charity, and hajj (pilgrimage). Traditional Islam includes spiritually based and healthy practices, such as prayer five times a day (early morning, noon, midafternoon, sunset, and evening), fasting, and prohibition against the consumption of pork products and intoxicating liquors. There are also prohibitions against gambling, sexual relations outside of marriage (but with the socially sanctioned tradition of having more than one wife given the lower ratio of men to women), and behavior or dress that is indecent. There are obvious health benefits for avoiding such high-risk behaviors as prescribed by Islamic tradition. Avoiding alcohol intoxication also helps prevent the disinhibition effects and the accompanying social problems. Avoiding pork would also provide protection against swine-related foodborne diseases, such as Salmonella typhimurium gastroenteritis, Yersinia enterocolitis; and viral illnesses from pork or pork products, including foot-and-mouth disease, classic swine fever (hog cholera), African swine fever, and swine vesicular viral disease.

Earlier, Jewish laws in the Old Testament forbid the consumption or touching the dead carcass of pigs, because they are "unclean to you" (Leviticus 11:7–8; Deuteronomy 14:8). This unclean description of pigs is consistent with their diet of eating dirt, urine, and fecal matter, decaying animals and vegetables, maggots, and cancerous growths off other animals. Pigs are also helpful for clearing an area of rattlesnakes, because they will eat the snakes and not be harmed by their venomous bites. Within a few days after being butchered, a pig's flesh quickly becomes a substrate for flies to lay eggs which hatch as larvae and fill the flesh with worms. Also, given their "unclean" diet and their inability to sweat or perspire, the meat and fat of pork can be 30 times more toxic than beef or venison. Pork is also digested more rapidly than beef or venison (4 hours versus 8–9 hours), resulting in a much higher level of toxins when it is consumed. Even the use of modern microwave ovens may fail to protect against pork-related illness such as salmonellosis. There may be no safe cooking temperature to ensure the killing of the dozens of parasites in pork, such as flukes, tapeworms, trichinae, and worms. Pork is not the only source of foodborne diseases, and such pathogens in general are emerging as a major public health challenge. Societies have developed some ways of preparing pork, vegetables, and other meats to help reduce the risks of foodborne illnesses by drying, smoking, salt- and sugar-curing, and of course cooking.

Fasting

Rumi, in the Middle Ages, stated that "being hungry is better than the maladies that come with satiety. Subtlety and lightness and being true to your devotion are some of the advantages of fasting."

During the lunar holy month of Ramadan, Muslims all over the world fast from sunrise to sunset. This fasting means abstaining completely from foods, drinks, and sexual intercourse from dawn to sunset. As stated in the Qur'an (2:183): "O ye who believe! Fasting is prescribed to you as it was prescribed to those before you, so that ye may learn self-restraint." Fasting is thought to purge the body of passion and sin and reduce the risk of disease. Once passion has been controlled, it is possible to clear the mind (an element of the spiritual body) of conscious thought. This allows the mystic to establish contact with saints, spirits, sources of magical power, and, ultimately, with Allah. Fasting also teaches patience and unselfishness, for when a person fasts, he or she can identify with the pains and deprivations of others less fortunate.

In naturopathic medicine, fasting is used as a method of detoxifying the body. It is a rapid way to increase the elimination of wastes within the body to facilitate healing. Also, a number of medical conditions have been treated with fasting, ranging from obesity, allergies, and chemical poisoning, to irritable bowel syndrome. Obesity is becoming epidemic within the United States. Further, intermittent fasting, caloric restriction, and undernutrition (but not malnutrition) have been associated with increased life span for both animals and humans. As suggested by Rumi, one of the results of overeating may be a shorter life.

Meditation

Rumi also stated that "when you neglect your meditation, you contract with pain. This is God's way of telling you that your inner pain can become visible. Don't ignore it."

Meditation is one of the most important Sufi ways for drawing nearer to Allah by "remembering" God and thus treating one's inner heart that has become distant, diseased, and hardened. (In a related way, paraphrasing Samuel Johnson (1709–1784), "mankind needs less to be instructed than to be reminded.") Worshipful meditation is an integral part of Sufism and is also known as "Divine Remembrance," Dhikr, or Zekr (Chishti 1991). As noted in the Qur'an: "Then do ye remember Me, I will remember you" (2:152). The place of worship or the Takiya is also known as the "House of Remembrance." These Sufi meditation practices are above and beyond the traditional prayers.

Such meditation practices involve a prescribed number of recitations of verses from the Qur'an using prayer beads (i.e., a rosary to keep count), such as "la illaha illa Allah," or "there is no god but Allah (The God)" (Ansha 1991), or other remembrances, such as "The Beautiful Names" of Allah. For some tariqas (e.g., Tariqa Casnazaniyyah), this recitation is done aloud with accompanying head movements symbolizing a hammer slamming the heart that has become "hardened like a stone." The remoteness from Allah causes this hardness, and the remembrance is the remedy. As noted in the Qur'anic verse 2:74, "Thenceforth were your hearts hardened: they became like a rock and even worse in hardness." Other tariqas use silent remembrances or use different movements altogether. Meditation has been suggested to help treat diseases.

It has been suggested that the number of recitations to treat diseases end with a zero (e.g., 100, 200, 300) (Chishti 1991). Again, from the Sufi perspective, worshipful meditation is a means of drawing near to Allah, and with that connection may come transcendent events.

Research has documented the many health and physiological benefits of meditation, including decreasing blood pressure, rate of breathing, heart rate, and oxygen consumption. The positive effects of meditation are associated with the production of a physiological "relaxation response" that is opposite to the "fight-or-flight response" (see Chapter 6). Thus the regular meditative practice of Sufism may also contribute to improved health.

Prayer

Prayers of Salat (the Arabic term) are performed five times a day by Muslims throughout the world. For these prayers all Muslims face the Kaaba in Mecca, which is believed to have been built by the Prophet Abraham. These five prayers are done at dawn, noon, mid-afternoon, sunset, and nightfall and can be done anywhere, but community prayer at the mosque on Fridays also serves the function, as with other religious traditions, of bringing the community together with all the health benefits of social support. Hygiene or ablution is a traditional part of Muslim prayers, known as Wudu. This practice of hand washing was done routinely many centuries before the discovery of germs and antisepsis. It is interesting to note that although it has been very much a part of religion and ceremony, hygiene was very slow to come to the practice of Western medicine and met with much resistance (see Chapters 1 and 2).

Today the health benefits of good hygiene practices are the standard of care. In addition to hygiene, the healing benefits of prayer are now becoming recognized within the disciplines of science and medicine (Dossey 1996, 2001). "Prayer works. More than 130 controlled laboratory studies show, in general, that prayer or a prayer like state of compassion, empathy, and love can bring about healthful changes in many types of living things, from humans to bacteria. This does not mean prayer always works, any more than drugs and surgery always work, but that, statistically speaking, prayer is effective" (Dossey 1996).

The psychology of Sufi

The notion of the heart and the ego or lower self (Arabic, *nafs*, see Chapter 8) has played a prominent role in Sufi psychology

(Ansha 1991; Chishti 1991). The spiritual path of Sufism is geared toward inner spiritual development by helping the follower in the purification or extinction (*fana*) of the ego/lower self (*nafs*) or more basic appetitive aspects of the body and selfish and mean-spirited desires. The health benefits of a system that helps manage the excessive appetitive motives would have positive implications for a number of disorders of overindulgence, such as weight problems and addictions. Disorders of excess are significant causes of morbidity within the West, with obesity one of the most serious threats.

The heart, in Sufism, is related to one's spiritual self. As mentioned earlier, the head movement that accompanies the recitation meditation, Dhikr practice, symbolizes a hammer slamming the heart that has become a stone so that its true luster can shine through. It is within the heart or inner being that spiritual development and battles occur. This internal battleground is the true concept of jihad.

Jihad

One of the often misunderstood concepts in Islam is the term "Jihad," usually associated with the notion of "holy war" and terrorism. The definition of Jihad from the Qur'an means "exerting the best efforts," or some type of "struggle" and "resistance," to achieve some goal (Fatoohi 2002), somewhat akin to the karma yoga path of Chapter 5. The Qur'an discusses two types of jihad, "peaceful jihad" and "armed jihad." Armed jihad was permitted as a temporary response for Muslims against armed aggression. The early Muslim community lived fourteen years under the guidance of the revelations made to Muhammad before they were given permission to fight back to defend themselves. Fourteen years of peace followed by fourteen centuries of conflicts. The Qur'an uses a different term, *qital*, when referring to fighting an enemy. It is also forbidden in Islam to take an innocent life, because killing one innocent person is like killing the whole group, and, conversely, saving one person is like saving the whole community (Qur'an 5:32).

Peaceful jihad, however, is the permanent struggle in which every Muslim must continuously exert efforts against evil desires within the lower self. Such an ongoing inner struggle uses such facilities as intuition to allow oneself to overcome lower drives and draw nearer to Allah, with all the spiritual, material, and metaphysical benefits.

Afflictions

One of the greatest challenges people currently face in the world is trying to understand and endure personal crises, illness, and afflictions. The Islamic and Sufi perspective holds that whatever happens to an individual occurs only by the will of Allah. One might ask, however, "Why would Allah allow bad things to happen to people?"

Affliction brings people closer to God. Thus, affliction teaches humility, patience, and thankfulness from Allah. It is our lower self that rebels against Allah during afflictions, and distances us from the source of needed help. The psychology of human behavior is keenly noted in the Qur'an (C:4) where people tend to "boast in prosperity, and curse in adversity." Faith in the oneness of Allah, and enduring these struggles, is the heart of peaceful jihad and brings one closer to the God.

Faith

Faith has also been suggested as an important factor in the psychology of healing from a Sufi perspective, as in other healing traditions. Illnesses can be treated in many ways, but no matter how many different treatments are used, they may still fail to heal the patient. In order for a treatment to work, first, even if the patient does not have faith in God, he must have faith in the doctor and in whatever treatment he suggests. Second, the doctor who is performing the treatment must have faith in God; he must have God's qualities, His love, and His patience. The doctor must give all responsibility to God, instead of thinking that he is the one who is responsible for curing the patient.

When these conditions exist, when the patient has faith in the doctor, and the doctor has faith in God, then treatment becomes very easy, and the illness will be cured, at least to a certain extent. The physiology by which faith heals has been studied through the placebo effect. Any treatment works better when the patient and doctor both believe in the treatment, and when the patient believes in the doctor. And all treatments work better when they meet cultural expectations.

Healing

Although the primary focus of Sufism is on attainment to Allah, some Sufis have developed a particular focus on healing—as in Budhism in Tibet, where all monks engage in devotional practices, and some focus on healing. Often there is a blend of Sufi philosophy with other healing traditions, as well as incorporation of the use of herbs, food, and other practices (Chishti 1991).

The Sufi Healing Order offers both training and services in spiritual healing. Some healing services are conducted within a group prayer circle. Members also visit ill persons, offering spiritual support.

Far eastern islands of Indonesia

Sufi philosophy has played a major role in influencing traditional medical practices in the Indonesian island of Java. Indonesia was swept by the further reach of Islam in the fifteenth century extending eastward to the island of Timor and northeast to the southern Philippines. The earlier Vedic influences of Further India were swept back to the island of Bali where they can be observed today.

The Javanese medical system draws on a wide variety of symbols, roles, and interactional patterns, none of which are strictly medical. Concepts of personal identity, cosmology, power and knowledge are blended into a body of closely related theories explaining the origins of disease and motivating highly diverse treatment strategies. Medical pluralism is an inherent feature of Javanese traditional medicine. There are two primary modes of medical practice. One, practiced by Sufi *wali* (holy men), is based on Islamic mystical concepts of miracles and gnosis. The other, practiced by *dukun* (curers), involves the use of morally suspect forms of magical power.

These two modes of medical practice can be seen to reflect a cosmological divide between light and dark, or in religious terms, between Islam and animism.

Spiritual healing

Western religious traditions have provided intercessory prayer and distant healing intercessions, and organized Christian churches harbor charimastic movements for the expression of this kind of faith and healing. Daniel Benor, a practicing holistic psychiatrist, addressed the evidence-based question of spiritual healing:

> "Does spiritual healing work? Does research confirm that healing is an effective therapy?" An impressive number of studies with excellent design and execution answer this question with a "Yes." If we take a broad view, out of 191 controlled experiments of healing…close to two thirds (64.9 percent) of all the experiments demonstrate significant effects. (Benor 2001)

Spiritual healing effects can be demonstrated on animals, plants, single-celled organisms, bacteria, yeasts, and DNA. Similarly, medical research is demonstrating that devices producing pulsing magnetic fields of particular frequencies can stimulate the healing of a variety of tissues. Therapists from various schools of energy medicine can project, from their hands, fields with similar frequencies and intensities. Research documenting these different approaches as efficacious is mutually validating. One common denominator appears to be the pulsating magnetic field, called a biomagnetic field when it emanates, for example, from the hands of a therapist.

Rapid healing

One healing phenomenon from the Middle East that has received little attention from the West (probably for geographical and political reasons) is the spiritual practice of rapid wound healing from "deliberately caused bodily damage" (DCBD). This phenomenon is also seen through South and Southeast Asia particularly among Hindu populations. At a major Sufi school, the extraordinary phenomenon of instantaneous wound healing from DCBD is cultivated. Followers (dervishes) of this Sufi school have been observed to demonstrate instantaneous healing of DCBD. For example, dervishes have inserted a variety of sharp instruments (e.g., spikes, skewers) into their body, hammered daggers into the skull bone and clavicle, and chewed and swallowed glass and sharp razor blades without harm to the body, and with complete control over pain, bleeding, and infection, as well as rapid wound healing—within 4 to 10 seconds. Researchers report that such extraordinary abilities are accessible to anyone, and not restricted to only a few talented individuals who have spent years in special training. These unusual healing phenomena have also been reproduced under controlled laboratory conditions and are not similar to hypnosis.

Similar observations of DCBD phenomena have been observed in various parts of the world in a variety of religious and nonreligious contexts. For example, trance surgeons in Brazil have employed sharp instruments to cut, pierce, or inject substances into a patient's body for therapeutic purposes. Laboratory electroencephalogram (EEG) investigation of trance surgeons has shown that this "state of spirit possession" for the healers was associated with a hyperaroused brain state (waves in the 30–50-Hz band). Unfortunately, besides little scientific attention being given to the investigation of these rapid healing claims in the United States, such claims for extraordinary healing abilities have been met with scorn and have even been challenged by so-called skeptic groups, such as the Committee for the Scientific Investigation of Claims of the Paranormal (CSCIOP). These groups offer monetary incentives to discredit such claims in unscientific and dangerous settings (Mulacz 1998; for a discussion and response, see Dossey 2001; Fatoohi and Al-Dargazelli 1999).

Followers of this Sufi school describe the ability to accomplish DCBD as an "others-healing phenomena" within the context of healing energies. This "higher energy" is alleged to be instantly transferable, mediated through the shaikh from Allah, and is reminiscent of the principle of non-locality in "spooky" modern physics (Chapters 1 and 2).

These systematic observations lay the foundation for more traditional laboratory followup studies that can be conducted with what Thomas Kuhn, in *The Structure of Scientific Revolutions* (Kuhn 1970), might call the puzzle-solving process of "normal science." Kuhn notes that anomalous observations that do not fit within existing paradigms can result in a crisis that may lead to the revolutionary process of a paradigm shift. Normal science in general has long been criticized for lack of interest in translating basic science into practical applications.

A demonstration of such rapid wound healing within a Western medical setting has great scientific implications. If such spiritually based healing approaches are genuine, they hold much promise for addressing some of today's most serious medical issues.

The investigation of such unusual healing phenomena in the West raises many questions. What should be measured within a scientific context? Would standard measures of brain and immune activity be associated with changes in rapid wound healing, or should standard measures, such as EEG activity, be used in less standard ways? Would high-frequency EEG activity need to be examined for hyperaroused brain states? Would new approaches be needed to detect "fields of consciousness," such as the examination of changes in the output from a "random event generator"? Here we see that Sufism, through this rapid healing phenomenon, joins Ayurveda, Unani, Yoga, and Tibetan medicine in suggesting that a non-local "consciousness" is ultimately the seat of the mysterious healing powers that have become familiar through their centuries of routine use, mediated by hundreds of generations of healers, on literally millions of people.

Work in this field takes us beyond Newton's classical mechanics to quantum mechanics and quantum physics to account for possible subtle energy constructs. Eric Leskowitz (2005) proposes a multidimensional model of wound healing to incorporate energy concepts and help shift our current paradigm of wound healing, and healing in general, beyond the physical and psychological dimensions, or as he describes it, from biology to spirit. How does Sufism explain it?

Sufism can provide a unified theory for mechanistic, mind-body, and spiritual healing. Traditional Islamic theology recognizes that Allah (God) created a world that can apparently operate under mechanistic and Newtonian principles at the level of everyday experience. Thus, there is no rejection of mechanistic views from traditional Islamic philosophy. Sufi philosophy goes further, noting that mechanistic views can also be explained within a vitalistic perspective. From this point of view, Sufism can account for both mechanistic and energy-based rapid healing phenomena in ways that Newtonian models of modern biomedicine cannot explain.

Thus, most of the time the world operates by mechanical laws, but mediation by a Sufi Shaikh (based on the Shaikh's nearness to, and through, Allah, in the view of Islam) would allow "for fire not to burn" or a "knife not to cut," thus suspending mechanistic laws. The Qur'an is clear in several verses that so-called natural laws can be suspended by Allah.

Nearer, my God, to thee

The goal of the Sufi and all spiritual paths is nearness to God. In Sufism, this goal is achieved by following the Sufi path and practices, and by jihad, or by struggling against the lower self or nafs. It is the lower self that keeps humans distant from God. Islam and Sufism are about surrendering to the will of God through following this path. Once near God, alterations of mechanistic laws may occur. This nearness to Allah is the explanation for "miracles" performed within religious contexts of ancient times and today.

Sufism teaches that the heart is the center of being, and that it becomes diseased. It becomes hardened (as in the case of the ancient Egyptian Pharoah of the book) from wrong acts (sins). Sufism offers healing for the heart, as noted in the Qur'an: "O mankind! There hath come to you a direction from your Lord and a healing for the (diseases) in your hearts—and for those who believe a guidance and a Mercy" (10:57). When the heart has been purified, through jihad, true healing will occur.

Energy and unity

Sufism is a mystical tradition within Islam based on drawing nearer to Allah through the spirituality of Muhammad and his sacerdotal descendants. Masters of present Sufi schools trace their origins back to him through a chain of Masters. Sufism can be described as a path or way of attainment to Allah, with associated paranormal experiences, knowledge, and healing. The Sufi way involves following orthodox Islamic practices such as daily prayer, fasting, and some dietary prohibition, as well as frequent worshipful meditation. These practices have not only spiritual purposes, but also many positive health implications that help keep body and soul integrated.

Although Sufism generally is focused on spiritual development, some Sufi schools have focused on healing. This healing is a blend of Sufi philosophy with other Islamic healing traditions. Paranormal Sufi healing abilities have been observed and explained on the basis of a spiritual link mediated through the Sufi Master back to Muhammad and Allah. Such phenomena from the Sufi way do not appear, scientifically, to result from meditative or altered states of consciousness, but may be the result of a higher, non-local consciousness.

An implication of Sufism for health lies in the fact that Western high-tech medicine can be helpful for medical and surgical emergencies, but may not be as helpful for chronic non-life-threatening conditions. What is needed for healing lies beyond "high tech," in "high touch." Sufism is one of the least studied approaches that offer an integration of the spiritual dimensions of healing.

The Sufi way is among the universal paths of spiritual traditions, including prayer, fasting, and meditation and ultimate attainment of nearness to god (Allah).

As noted in a book by Michael Jawer, the *Spiritual Anatomy of Emotion* (Jawer with Micozzi 2009), Larry Dossey (2001) originally anticipated the need for the return of spirituality to medicine in 2001 at the turn of the new millennium:

> Modern medicine has become [one of the] spiritually malnourished professions in our society. Because we have thoroughly disowned the spiritual component of healing,

most healers throughout history would view our profession today as inherently perverse. They would be aghast at how we have squeezed the life juices and the heart out of our calling. Physicians have spiritual needs like anyone else, and we have paid a painful price for ignoring them. It simply does not feel good to practice medicine as if the only thing that matters were the physical; something feels left out and incomplete. (Dossey 2001)

Among the traditions of India, Tibet, and the Middle East, we saw that Tibetan medicine is most closely aligned with the ideals, and ultimately the practice, of Buddhism, a non-theistic approach to understanding the flow of vital energy in the universe. Sufism represents a theistic approach to such understanding that is almost uniquely aligned with pure spirit and can be seen in the active devotion of the Sufi "whirling dervishes." Anyone who has had the privilege to witness them in action cannot help but feel the energy in the room. In Asia, ancient medicine originated in magical-religious practices, and then added the physical modalities and materials (alchemical and herbal remedies) of healing. With modern interpretations of fundamental science, as evidenced in Maharishi Ayurveda and Sufism, for example, there is room to restore the spiritual aspects of universal consicousness to the healing equation. If Sufi embodies pure spirit, it takes us on the historic quest back to the origins of Nature and the cosmos itself.

Chapter 10

Conclusion

Ethnomedicine of Vital Energy

We hope this book has opened a door to understanding the health beliefs and behaviors of traditional societies in the Middle Asian region of the globe. The concept of a "vital energy" is a common feature of health and healing through time in this place. The West has generally become familiar with how the concept of *qi* animates, informs and guides medicine in China, or East Asia, the "Greater China" of antiquity. This book shows how this same idea of a vital energy is central to medicine in India, Tibet, the Middle East and Middle Asia—or the "Further India" of antiquity, as well. We have also introduced how the roots of energy medicine were introduced to thinking in Europe, Colonial England, and Early America—culminating in a Western tradition of contemplation and meditative practice, together with home grown traditions, and ultimately giving rise to new concepts in modern physical science about the fundamental character of the cosmos itself.

Vital energy and flow in Middle Asian medicine

When considering the ancient medical traditions of China, India, Tibet, and the Middle East, it is useful to recognize that all of South, East, and Southeast Asia came under the influence of two of the earliest civilizations at the dawn of history. The cultural diffusion concepts of "Further India" and "Greater China" are useful to consider as succeeding waves of influence emanating out from the great river valleys of the Indus and Yellow River, respectively, carrying along common discoveries and understandings of the nature of human life and health. One may view the outgrowth of Buddhism from the Hindu Prince Guatama (the Buddha) as a manifestation of a wave of influence from "Further India," which gave birth to the next waves in Tibet and Greater China. Ultimately one may see a third wave, of Islam, during the seven hundred years from 750 to 1450 CE, spread ideas from the western border of North Africa to the eastern edge of Indonesia, which carried along ancient Greco-Roman (Unani, or Arabic for "Greek") concepts of health and healing which it had incorporated and preserved following the Classical Era in the West. All three of these traditions place emphasis on the concept of vital energy as central to health and healing. Just as vital energy itself flows, so has the very concept of a vital energy in healing flowed throughout this region for centuries.

This concept of vital energy (*prana* in India, and *qi* in China) is found to be fundamental in many Asian medical traditions. In the West, *qi* has been translated to imply the flow of energy, spirit, or breath that animates living beings. Ancient Chinese ideograms depicted the term with three strokes to symbolize cloudlike vapor, as when the breath is seen on a cold day. The evanescent nature of the concept of *qi* has been difficult to capture in translation, or transliteration, and is perhaps best captured, at least partially, by comparisons among these global traditions.

The potency of energy to help (and to harm) healing finds one parallel in Western medicine by the placebo/nocebo dualism, and the "words that heal/words that harm" concept of Dr. Larry Dossey (1993).

A few (more) words about Chinese medicine

While this book focuses on vital healing in India, Tibet, and the Middle East, we continue to utilize the concepts of energy and flow in the analysis of *qi* in Chinese medicine specifically. It is striking how all of Chinese medicine, energy anatomy, and pathology use terms relating to the political governance of society as metaphors for how the human body is regulated—essentially as a description of human physiology. This metaphor is striking to the Western reader, since Western biomedicine uses the metaphor of a machine to describe functions of the human body. While the human body has been used as a metaphor for the political governance of a human society by Thomas Hobbes in his famous treatise, *Leviathan* (1651), we do not observe the reverse application in Western medicine. Leviathan was, in fact, the body politic made visible—a social body composed of cells of individual men, just as the human body is composed of individual cells.

Modern medicine is largely based on the fact that, essentially, the body is made up of populations of cells comprising tissues and organs that work together as regulated by physiology, just as populations of individuals make up societies that work together under political governance. So, the metaphors of Chinese medicine are another useful way of representing human functional anatomy and physiology. As an empirical system, Chinese medicine is tremendously sophisticated and nuanced, in terms of devising treatments tailored to each individual and his or her specific conditions.

The Chinese use of metaphors in medicine that describe human physiology in terms that come from human socio-political organization may relate to the preoccupation of Chinese civilization with the Emperor, his Mandarins, and the bureaucratic organization that provided the foundation for government administration of complex works and operations. The modern biomedical system is not so different in the West, with the Emperor and Mandarins of medicine regularly holding court at the National Institutes of Health, for example.

One of the great projects of the ancient Chinese civilization that at once created and sustained it, was the construction of canals or "waterways" for irrigation agriculture and for transportation. The organization of labor for such projects had a transactional relationship to the development of Chinese social organization and political control. These processes and relationships were described by Karl Wittfogel (1963) in the classic treatise *Oriental Despotism*. The inherent relations of the contours of Chinese society with major public "infrastructure" projects, the political organization of the Chinese government, and the Chinese pictographic language used for communications resulted in a rich vocabulary of metaphors used in describing medical aspects of the human body: waterways, or channels, in the original Chinese language.

Western translations using words like "meridians" do not correctly map to the Chinese metaphorical concepts. The chapters in this book provide a new map and guide for vital energy in other Asian traditions beyond *qi* in Chinese medicine.

Contemporary concerns and comparisons

During the twentieth century the terms of the discussion about energy and matter were changed by the fundamental discoveries of quantum physics. Experiments performed in the first quarter of the twentieth century indicated that subatomic particles, the supposed building blocks of nature, did not appear to be composed of solid matter. In some of these experiments, particles behaved as if they were waves. While the Nobel Prize had been awarded to nineteenth-century British physicist J. J. Thompson for his discovery that electrons are particles, a generation later it was awarded to his son George P. Thompson for *his* discovery that electrons are waves.

It was observed that electrons take instantaneous, discontinuous, quantum jumps from one atomic orbit to another, with no intervening time and no travel through space—an impossible act for a classic particle. It was shown that an individual subatomic particle cannot have both a precise position and a precise momentum simultaneously (the "uncertainty" principle of German quantum physicist Werner Heisenberg), a situation that could not apply to a solid material particle. It was also found that electrons can, with predictable regularity, tunnel through a solid barrier that, classically, would be impenetrable. Finally, it has been revealed that in a pair of subatomic particles, whatever is done to one affects the other, *immediately*, without time delay, without any detectable form of energy transfer or communication, and no matter how great the distance separating them. This is not a causal effect. Ths is a demonstration of *non-local connectivity*, or what has come to be called *entanglement*, which defies mechanistic and even relativistic assumptions. On the basis of these findings, the basic principles of quantum mechanics (often known as the Copenhagen Interpretation) modify a materialist worldview: (1) no solid matter (supported by the wave/particle paradox, quantum jumps, uncertainty, tunneling, and entanglement); (2) no strict causality(as precise predictions for individual subatomic particles are impossible); (3) no locality (quantum entanglement defies the strictly local connections of classic materialism); (4) no reductionism (because entanglement nullifies the view that there are isolated particles).

The Copenhagen Interpretation was not able to be put to experimental test for decades, leaving some physicists unconvinced that solidity, causality, locality, and reductionism had to be abandoned. During and despite World War I, German scientist Albert Einstein carried on a correspondence with British astronomer Arthur Eddington, leading Eddington with his Royal Astronomical Society colleague Frank Watson Dyson to conduct experiments during a total eclipse of the sun on the island of Principe in Africa in 1919, demonstrating that starlight is bent by the gravity of the sun, providing proof of Einstein's theory of relativity. By the 1980s, a number of different experiments produced results that consistently contradicted the theories of materialism (often called local realism) and consistently confirmed the predictions of quantum mechanics. These studies found that, once two particles have interacted, they are instantaneously entangled, correlated non-locally, over arbitrarily vast distances—an impossibility in materialism.

These results do not invalidate materialism altogether. In the everyday world of "large" objects, the mechanistic causation of Newtonian physics is approximately correct, which is why much of medicine has been able to rely on it. However, contemporary

Western medicine has not incorporated into its perspectives on health and healing these many clues and observations from fundamental physics about the nature of reality. Thus, Western society has advanced into the twenty first century using modern cutting edge technologies guided by nineteenth century theories of materialist physics (and typological biology).

At the fundamental, subatomic level, materialism conflicts both with theory and with frequently replicated experimental evidence. This conflict gives rise to a fundamentally different worldview. Many physicists now argue that nature is composed of probability waves that are a function of intelligence or "consciousness" alone, not of discrete physical particles—leading Eddington and others to an understanding that "the stuff of the universe is mind stuff." The equations of quantum mechanics may ultimately be describing a world made of abstract patterns of intelligence.

In view of these uniformly idea-like characteristics of the quantum-physical world, the proper answer to the question, "What sort of world do we live in?" would seem to be: "We live in an idea-like world, not a matter-like world." There is, in fact, in the quantum universe no natural place for matter. This conclusion, curiously, is the exact reverse of the circumstance that in the classic physical universe there was not a natural place for mind.

In quantum field theory, the probability wave for a particle is described as a fluctuation in an underlying, nonmaterial field (known as a force field or matter field). Furthermore, in recent superunified theories, physicists have described all the force and matter fields that make up the universe as modes of vibration of one underlying, unified field, sometimes called the superfield or superstring field. All the order and intelligence of the laws of nature arise from this one fundamental, nonmaterial field, as does all matter. Not only are particles really just waves, but also those waves ultimately are made of an underlying field, as ocean waves are "made of" ocean water. Returing to the metaphor of water, and waterways or channels, theory and research on *qi*, as well as observations from contemporary practices of energy medicine may be seen in this new light.

Health and healing in our time

Different fields of scholarly study, academic approaches, and clinical practices have been divided by somewhat arbitrary boundaries placed upon expertise, knowledge, and specialization. However, insights from different fields have been converging on a new, central understanding of energy in human physiology as related to health and healing. Aspects of energy have been central to ethnomedical practices in the East. In the West, clinical fields as diverse as Biosynthesis, Cardiology, Immunology, Kinesiology, Psychology, and Therapeutic Touch have all given rise to medical treatments using the energetic aspects of human physiology that are perhaps best understood under the principles of fundamental physics. That so many different approaches using different clinical tools can influence the energy of the body demonstrates that vital energy is inherent to the nature of human physiology. These insights have led us to the threshold of a new era for a more complete kind of health and healing in the twenty-first century. Ancient wisdom about health and healing is a treasure trove of understanding, as well as practical applications, for a more complete, healthier longer and more human life.

Some very practical guidelines are provided for avoiding and managing several of the most common medical problems of our modern society in the Appendix while avoiding side effects and complications (and costs).

Appendix

Ancient Wisdom for Modern Healing

There are remedies available from the ancient wisdom of Middle Asian medicines that are useful for many of today's common medical problems. Secrets derived directly from the ancient Sanskrit texts of Ayurveda are provided here for *allergies* and *asthma, arthritis, cancer, fever, headache, high blood pressure,* and peptic *ulcer* that can help prevent the development of these disorders and provide relief for those already suffering from these medical conditions. If you suffer from these disorders, have family members who do, or a family history of them, these secrets offer real alternatives to you and your loved ones.

Furthermore, they offer help without the risks of side effects and complications that are unfortunately so common with the high-powered drugs, surgery and medical procedures of mainstream treatments. And beyond, these remedies also offer natural enhancements that will generally improve your quality of *life, longevity,* and probably your *relationships* with your fellow human beings.

As we said at the beginning of this book, because these approaches treat the causes and not just the symptoms of diseases, they are effective at *preventing* as well as *treating* these problems. In addition to what is offered here, ancient Sanskrit remedies are available for many other medical problems, such as *diabetes mellitus*, and *viral hepatitis*, but require treatment with complex herbal preparations (available today from trusted sources) that are beyond the scope of this book.

Allergies and asthma

Astyma is the Sanskrit term for allergies, from which the English word asthma is derived. Ayurveda views allergies as altered reactivity caused by weakened metabolism in one or more of the seven tissues of the body. They are categorized according to the three constitutional types: vata, pitta and kapha.

Immediate allergic reactions (*anaphylactic* reactions, from the Greek *ana-* meaning not or without and *phylaxis* meaning defense or protection) are seen as related to pitta. *Intermittent* allergies (pets, foods) are vata-pitta, or vata-kapha type, and delayed allergies (seasonal) are kapha.

Vata allergic symptoms include aches and pains, coughing, gas, sneezing and sensitivity to dirt, dust and pollens. Symptoms may also include heart palpitations, muscle allergies and wheezing (a symptom associated with the constriction of the airways found in asthma). People having these vata-type allergies may find they are sensitive to plants from the *Solanacea* family, for example, eggplant, potato, tomato, and deadly nightshade (the source of the drug atropine, or *bella donna*, from the Italian meaning "beautiful woman," because women during the 1700s, a time when Italy was a "fashion capital" of Europe, placed atropine in their eyes to cause dilation of the pupils, producing a "doe-eyed" look, due to the toxic effects on the autonomic nervous system affecting the ciliary muscles of the eyes). Other vata-type food sensitivities may include black beans, chick peas (garbanzo beans, for making houmus) and other beans. These allergies can often be managed with a vata-pacifying diet and vata-reducing herbs.

Pitta-type allergic symptoms include acne, contact dermatitis, eczema and sensitivity to heat and light, insect bites, foam (as in pillows and mattresses), formaldehyde and preservatives. Food sensitivities include bananas, eggs, carrots, grapefruit, garlic, pork, onions, and certain cheeses and spicy foods. A pitta-pacifying diet and herbs are recommended.

Kapha-type allergies include allergic rhinitis, asthma, hay fever and pollen sensitivities, and latent spring fever, causing symptoms of colds, runny nose and teary eyes, as well as laryngeal edema (swelling of the throat), and possibly generalized edema. Food sensitivities may include avocado, bananas, beef, cucumbers, dairy, lamb, lemons, peanuts, pork, and watermelon. A kapha-reducing diet with hot, green teas (with methyl xanthenes, such as caffeine and theophylline, which are natural treatments for decongestion and expansion of airways) and herbal teas are recommended.

The thymus gland and spleen are seen in Ayurveda as important to the immune system. In fact the thymus gland which is active in childhood and shrinks at adulthood is important in development of the "T-cell" lymphocytes, or white blood cells as part of the immune system; while the spleen has an important role in filtering the blood and houses large numbers of white blood cells, as well as a reserve of red blood cells. The *heating* factor of the thymus helps to maintain immunity in proper balance, and weakness may be a cause of kapha-type allergy. The spleen is understood as the *root* of the blood-forming system of the body and as a reservoir for blood (indeed it has this role during fetal development and early childhood, and acts as a reserve for blood cells during adulthood). The spleen also is said to contain components that destroy foreign particles and microbes, which is indeed an important function of the spleen as part of the immune system.

Weakness in the spleen is detectable in the pulse and likely to be present in individuals prone to allergies.

Arthritis

Arthritis is known as *amavata* in Sanskrit which implies the involvement of *ama* in the digestion and the vata dosha (wind). No distinction is made between rheumatoid arthritis (rheumatism), and osteo-degenerative arthritis. The cause is seen as all factors leading to poor digestion, with formation of ama: poor digestive function, excessive intake of fatty foods and meats, insufficient exercise and generally unhealthy foods and habits. In arthritis, ama is said to build up and leave the digestive tract, spilling over and accumulating in the joints and the heart (which are indeed involved in acute rheumatic fever). As implied by the name, vata is the principal dosha affected, aggravation of which causes indigestion, joint pain and rough skin. If pitta is also involved, a burning sensation may spread throughout the body especially in the joints (like some of the complaints in the mysterious modern syndromes of chronic fatigue and fibromyalgia, thought to be a rheumatoid illness). If kapha is further involved, the victim gradually becomes crippled. Less pain is experienced in the morning because at that time, ama is just beginning to move.

Treatments involved using diet, herbal remedies, and physical modalities and procedures to reduce ama and alleviate vata. The first line of treatment is as follows:

- mild fasting
- herbs with bitter taste, hot potency, and pungent, post-digestive after-taste for stimulation of the digestion (bitter-tasting herbs stimulate release of bile from the gall bladder into the intestines—a powerful digestant)
- sweating.

The second line then proceeds to the formal purification therapy of *Panchakarma*:

- preparation with oleation (oil treatments) and sweating
- comprehensive, five-part, classic purification therapy protocol over five days, including enema, herbal decoctions, and oil.

Third, the patient should then adopt a healthy regimen:

- avoid sleep during the day and after meals (to help stimulate digestion)
- avoid heavy foods
- regular massage.

Modern medical research has also shown the importance of *meditation* and *yoga* at increasing movement and reducing symptoms in arthritis. These steps are also generally helpful at preventing the development of arthritis. Effective ongoing treatments of arthritis, including childhood arthritic conditions (juvenile arthritis), involve wet massages in conjunction with enemas for digestion and detoxiciation. Affected joints can be given *tapotment* (massage term for light tapping or patting) with a cloth bag filled with rice cooked with milk and herbs—delivering heat and physical therapy to the joints. Simple massage with oils is also helpful.

There is no denying the benefits of these approaches for arthritis. One of the reasons that Western biomedicine is so often ineffective at treating arthritis may be related to missing the insight into the digestive system, and missing the connection to *diet* and *digestion* (or the rheumatologist sending the patient to the gastro-enterologist, and never "putting it together"). The importance of *exercise* and *physical activity* may or may not be addressed, and ignoring the importance of *sleep* patterns can generally be assumed, in Western medicine.

Cancer

There is no Sanskrit equivalent for the word cancer in classic Ayurveda. This omission may be consistent with findings from paleopathology that demonstrate the exceeding rarity, in prehistoric and ancient times, of most of today's common cancers (Micozzi 1991, 2007). If cancer did not exist to any appreciable extent in ancient Sanskrit civilization, the opportunities to describe it in cultural terms would not present themselves. Nonetheless, as fundamental metabolic disruption is evident in cancer (*cachexia*), there are Ayurvedic approaches to restoring metabolic balance in cancer *patients*, cancer *survivors*, and those at high *risk* of developing cancer due to *family history* or *genetics*. Ayurveda also recognizes the importance of the immune system here, which is seen as critical in modern cancer studies of the "immune surveillance" theory of cancer.

Under the influence of cancer, the three doshas function to destroy, rather than to preserve and nourish, the body. Vata causes normal cells to proliferate and become cancerous; pitta steals nutrients away from other tissues to feed cancer cells; and kapha allows these cancer cells to continue multiplying unchecked. Although it affects all three, it usually begins by dominating one of the doshas. This imbalance, together with accumulation of ama toxins and inadequate digestive function or fire sets the stage for cancer to appear.

Further, as a mind-body medicine, Ayurveda recognizes the intimate connection between suppressed *emotion* and suppressed immunity—another contributor to development and spread of cancer. Other factors recognized by Ayurveda include *devitalized* foods, chemical and radiation exposure long-term (which, or course, is itself the typical "*treatment*" of cancer in Western biomedicine), sedentary lifestyle, and even a lack of *spiritual* purpose in Life.

Because ama toxins are seen as the primary problem in cancer, of course, the classic detoxification therapy of *Panchakarma* is applied as the primary treatment. Patients are also given potent blood-cleansing herbs, immune strengthening herbs, circulatory stimulants, and special dosha-dispelling herbs according to the types of cancer. These Ayurvedic remedies have been subjected to testing in the laboratory which demonstrates effects at immune stimulation and re-differentiation of cancer cells literally back to normal cells (in distinction to Western chemotherapy which is entirely based on "cytotoxicity" or killing cancer cells, which harm all normal cells as well). These therapies are monitored clinically according to the patients skin tone and color (not the grey of chemotherapy patients), general demeanor among the other diagnostic procedures available in Ayurveda. In addition, remedies are given by dosha type, together with the anti-cancer herbs:

- *vata*: fresh ginger

- *pitta*: aloe gel

- *kapha*: honey and black pepper.

Headache

The common complaint of headache (or head pain; Sanskrit, *Shira Shula*), according to Ayurveda, has many different causes, including cold and flu, indigestion, lack of sleep, muscle tension, overwork and stress. *Migraine* headache specifically is thought to relate to inborn constitutional factors and are most commonly caused by vata and/or pitta imbalances.

Diagnosis is based upon the presence of symptoms associated with each of the three doshas.

- *Vata*: extreme pain, constipation, dry skin, and depression and anxiety; worsens with excessive activity, irregular lifestyle, stress and worry.

- *Pitta*: anger, burning sensation, irritability, light sensitivity, redness of eyes and face, nosebleeds; may be accompanied by liver problems or blood toxicity.

- *Kapha*: dull ache, heaviness, fatigue; may be accompanied by excess phlegm and salivation, or nausea and vomiting, or lung problems; accumulation of kapha in the head.

Treatments for both general headache and migraine are similar.

Sinus and congestive headaches (vata and kapha types) are usually associated with allergies, common colds and coughs due to colds. They are given decongestant and expectorant herbs:

- angelica, bayberry, calamus, ginger and wild ginger.

Effective soothing volatile oils are provided by:

- camphor, holy basil (also as tea), eucalyptus, tulsi, wintergreen.

In addition, therapies are added depending upon the dosha type:

- *vata*: purgation, herbal sedatives for restorative sleep
- *pitta*: liver cleansing with aloe powder or rhubarb root, cooling the head with sandalwood oil and avoiding heat and sun, internal gotu kola, inhalation of aromatic oils of rose or lotus.

Application of medicated oils to the head and in the nose are recommended for all forms of headache, including migraine.

Meditation and yoga are also helpful for tension headaches and migraine. In addition, Ayurvedic *Marma* therapy provides 107 points on the body which are sensitive to touch and may be stimulated to restore balance among the doshas. These points are accessed on the skin and specifically associated with enhancing immunity, raising serotonin levels, and increasing secretion of hormones associated with the pineal gland (the vestigial "third eye," sometimes associated with the *chakra* in the head). Five sets of points are specifically used in the treatment of headache:

- base of eyes (above the tear ducts, at the medial epicanthal folds)
- either side of the nose (one-third of the way down from bridge to nostrils)
- above the upper lip (mid-way between the margin of the upper lip and the base of the septum)

- top of the head (crown)
- at the pineal gland (third eye).

High blood pressure (hypertension)

Ayurveda understands both high venous blood pressure and arterial blood pressure (the latter typically measured as the "normal" 120/80 in Western medicine) because they both relate directly to the functioning of the heart and circulatory system. While high venous blood pressure (or congestion of the veins) is associated with heart failure (the typical congestive heart failure effectively treated with the herbally derived drug digitalis), this section addresses the arterial blood pressure elevation that is common and commonly known as hypertension in Western biomedicine.

Ayurveda considers it to be caused by imbalances in any of the three doshas:

- *Vata*: accumulation of toxins in digestive tract, absorbed into the blood, causing constriction of blood vessels:
  - rapid rise and fall in blood pressure ("labile hypertension"), accordingly, irregular heart rate and erratic pulse (as the heart responds to changes in blood pressure), dry tongue, insomnia, puffiness ("bags") under the eyes, constipation
  - primary treatments of colonic cleansing, medicated enemas
  - secondary vata-balancing diet of fish, fat-soluble vitamins A, D, E
  - garlic taken with milk.

- *Pitta*: toxins from poor digestion cause increased blood viscosity, redness of eyes, flushing of face, nosebleed, violent headache; anger, irritability, or burning sensation; sensitivity to light:
  - both systolic (first reading) and diastolic (second reading) pressures increased
  - treatment with bitter herbs, including aloe vera gel, bayberry, *Katuka*, and purgation

- ○ calming the mind with gotu kola, and other herbs to pacify pitta.

- *Kapha*: thought to originate in stomach, mucosal secretions produce elevated triglycerides and cholesterol, eventually contributing to atherosclerosis of the arteries:

  - ○ associated with edema, fatigue and hypothyroidism, obesity

  - ○ both systolic and diastolic pressures elevated, but diastolic may not rise as much as in pitta

  - ○ treated by elimination of dairy and fatty foods, and administration of herbs: cayenne (red) pepper, garlic, hawthorn berries, motherword, myrrh

  - ○ use of diuretics recommended only in kapha-type hypertension.

All three forms of *high blood pressure* are helped by:

- reduction of caffeine, salt, sugar and fatty and fried foods

- deep breathing exercises (the first step toward meditation)

- meditation and yoga daily (proven by modern research as effective and cost-effective without side effects, but many side benefits)

- moderate physical activity daily, for example, walking three miles.

Fever

Ayurveda sees fever (*Jvara Roga*) as both a disease and a symptom. We read in Chapter 1 that fever is simply a physiologic response by the body to arrest the multiplication of infectious disease-causing microbes, until the immune system can naturally overcome the infection (see Figure 1.1 on page 7). Accordingly, fever is viewed as a positive sign in Ayurveda because it is said to loosen and release ama, the cause of illness. It is often, therefore, allowed to run its course, letting the fever "break," unless one or more of the following danger signs are present:

- both high and prolonged elevation in body temperature

- history of prior seizure due to fever in a child
- rapid "depletion" of patient.

In addition to infection, causes are seen to be wrong combinations of food, for example, mixing hot with cold (fruit with starch, bananas with milk—a typical Western breakfast), excessive emotion such as anger or fear, stress from overwork. Fever is classified according to the three doshas:

- *Vata*: during vata time of day (dawn or dusk), or season (fall), begins in colon, pushes digestive fire into channels for transporting lymph, chyle and plasma, and heating the blood.
  - Primary: body ache, headache, shivering, tremors.
  - Secondary: backache, constipation, fatigue, insomnia.
- *Pitta*: midday and midnight, and during summer, onset like vata fever.
  - Primary: diarrhea, nausea and vomiting, rash, red eyes, perspiration, sensitivity to light.
  - Secondary: severed dehydration and reduction in blood pressure (fever with severe dehydration is typical of cholera, for example, which has been a historic problem in India and persists to this day in areas like Calcutta).

It may also be caused by alcohol abuse or very sour foods, or fermented beverages. Aspiring is not given because it may damage the stomach which is already involved in this condition.

- *Kapha*: morning and evening, and late winter and spring, production of excessive secretions which dampen digestive fires and causes undigested food to accumulate, increasing ama and forcing it out into the body.
  - Primary (prodromal): cold, congestion, runny nose.
  - Low grade fever, chest pain, cough, shortness of breath.
  - Laryngitis, sinusitis, sinus congestion, and sinus headache.

- ∘ Loss of appetite, cold and clammy skin, heavy and dull feeling.

Causes may be overexposure to cold, improper combinations of foods, especially involving milk.

Ayurveda is able to make further distinctions among fevers caused by intestinal parasites, and continuous versus fluctuating, or remittent, fevers (such as malaria, another historic problem in India).

Peptic ulcer (stomach and duodenum)

Peptic ulcers (*Parinama Shula*, in Ayurveda) are often associated with excess stomach acid and have been linked to the presence of specific bacteria in the stomach. Ulcers also appear in patients who have suffered shock, severe burns and head injuries. The following prodromal symptoms are addressed in Ayurvedic texts:

- belching of sour taste

- heartburn

- may be accompanied by nausea and vomiting.

Symptoms are brought on by overeating, alcohol, or greasy, sour or spicy foods. Hyperacidity may be accompanied by migraine headache.

Vomiting may alleviate symptoms. With a gastric ulcer, there is more pain between meals which is alleviated by eating and neutralizing excess acid. A duodenal ulcer is painful after eating as acidic stomach contents are emptied into the intestines.

Each of the three doshas are associated with stomach ulcers:

- *Vata*: excessive mental activity and nervousness lead to stress and overwork, causing ulcer; more gas in the stomach with radiating pain outward.

- *Pitta*: anger, aggression, frustration and anger cause high acid secretion in stomach and lead to ulcers; localized, sharp, penetrating pain, can cause waking in the middle of the night; more likely to lead to perforated ulcer.

- *Kapha*: deficiency of protective mucus secretions of stomach permit stomach acids to burn through the lining of the stomach, even in the presence of normal or low stomach acidity; deep, dull but bearable pain.

For all types of ulcers, a pitta-pacifying diet is given, excluding citrus, sour and spicy foods, and including ghee (clarified butter), milk and whole grains, such as basmati rice. Alcohol and smoking are avoided.

Specific herbal compounds are recommended before (*Avipattikara*) and after (*Jatamamsi, Kamadudha, Shatavari*) meals. For a bleeding ulcer, the remedy *Sat Isabgol* is taken with milk before sleep. If blood is seen passing into the stool (duodenal ulcer) other specific herbal remedies may be applied. Blood passing into the stool is a complicated sign. It occurs with bleeding from an ulcer but also with other dangerous conditions, such as bowel cancer, and should be referred to a medical doctor.

Find yourself and your medical profile according to Ayurveda

Use the information in this section on medical conditions with Tables A.1 to A.3. Which describes your type? Ayurvedic therapies are designed to rebalance and reintegrate the individual, based upon your type, and the type of the disorder from which you suffer or are at risk. Every remedy is seen as either *tonifying*, or nourishing, a deficiency or a weakness in the organ(s) involved, and/or to *detoxify*, or reduce, aggravation of the *doshas*. *Reducing* the specific problem usually comes first, followed by *rejeuvenation* to generally rebuild strength.

Reduction of the condition usually consists of *palliation*, followed by *purification*.

Palliation involves strengthening the digestive fires, reducing ama, and calming excess dosha. Purification involves the five-step classic therapy of *Panchakarma*.

All these approaches emphasize the natural, self-healing abilities of the patient while providing individually tailored treatments for the person and the disorder.

Table A.1 The three doshas: vata, pitta, kapha

Dosha	Effect of balanced dosha	Effect of imbalanced dosha	Factors aggravating
Vata	Exhilaration Clear and alert mind Perfect functioning of bowels Proper formation of all bodily tissues Sound sleep Excellent vitality and immunity Agitation or anger	Rough skin Weight loss Restlessness Constipation Decreased strength *Arthritis* Rheumatic disorder Cardiac arrhythmia Insomnia *Irritable bowel syndrome*	Excessive exercise Wakefulness Anxiety, worry Tuberculosis Suppression of natural urges Cold Fear or grief *Hypertension* Fasting Pungent, astringent, or bitter foods In Europe and USA: late autumn and winter In India: summer and rainy season
Pitta	Lustrous complexion Contentment Perfect digestion Softness of body Perfectly balanced heat and thirst mechanisms Balanced intellect	Yellowish complexion Excessive body heat Insufficient sleep Weak digestion Inflammation Inflammatory bowel diseases Skin diseases Heartburn *Peptic ulcer* Anger	Anger Strong sunshine Burning sensations Fasting Sesame products, linseed Yogurt Wine, vinegar Pungent, sour, or salty foods In Europe and USA: summer and early autumn In India: rainy season and autumn
Kapha	Strength Normal joints Stability of mind Dignity Affectionate, forgiving nature Strong and properly proportioned body Courage Vitality	Pale complexion Coldness Laziness, dullness Excessive sleep Sinusitis Respiratory diseases, *asthma* Excessive weight gain Loose joints Depression	Sleeping during daytime Heavy food Sweet, sour, or salty foods Milk products Sugar In Europe and USA: Spring In India: late winter and spring

Table A.2 Tastes and food qualities: effects on the doshas

Tastes	
Decrease vata	**Increase vata**
Sweet	Pungent
Sour	Bitter
Salty	Astringent
Decrease pitta	**Increase pitta**
Sweet	Pungent
Bitter	Sour
Astringent	Salty
Decrease kapha	**Increase kapha**
Pungent	Sweet
Bitter	Sour
Astringent	Salty
Major food qualities	
Decrease vata	**Increase vata**
Heavy	Light
Oily	Dry
Hot	Cold
Decrease pitta	**Increase pitta**
Cold	Hot
Heavy	Light
Oily	Dry
Decrease kapha	**Increase kapha**
Light	Heavy
Dry	Oily
Hot	Cold

Table A.3 Common examples of the six tastes and major food qualities

Six tastes and common examples
Sweet: sugar, milk, butter, rice, breads
Sour: yogurt, lemon, cheese
Salty: salt
Pungent: spicy foods, peppers, ginger, cumin
Bitter: spinach, other green leafy vegetables
Astringent: beans, pomegranate
Six major food qualities and common examples
Heavy: cheese, yogurt, wheat products
Light: barley, corn, spinach, apples
Oily: dairy products, fatty foods, oils
Dry: barley, corn, potato, beans
Hot: hot (temperature) foods and drinks
Cold: cold foods and drinks

Biographies

Mones Abu-Asab holds a Ph.D. degree in phylogenetic systematics from Ohio University, USA. Before joining the National Cancer Institute (NCI) in 1998, he taught at Birzeit University and worked on phylogenetic analysis at the Smithsonian Institution, vaccine analysis at Walter Reed Army Institute of Research, and ultrastructural pathology at George Washington University. He is currently an ultrastructural biologist at the Laboratory of Pathology of NCI.

Hakima Amri holds a PhD in reproductive physiology and steroid biochemistry from Pierre and Marie Curie University, Paris, France. She is the co-founder of the Complementary and Alternative Medicine (CAM) educational initiative at Georgetown University. Dr. Amri is the Director of the unique CAM Master of Science program in Physiology since its launch in 2003. Her research focuses on integrating evidence-based CAM to biomedical research.

Kevin Ergil, MA, MS, LAc, Diplomate in Oriental Medicine (NCCAOM), FNAAOM, FAAPM, is a Professor at the Finger Lakes School of Acupuncture and Oriental Medicine of NYCC. He is a practitioner of Traditional Chinese Medicine and a medical anthropologist. He has served as a director of the Society for Acupuncture Research and as a member of the advisory board. He is a past president of the American College of Traditional Chinese Medicine, San Francisco, and was the founding Dean of the Pacific College of Oriental Medicine, New York Campus. He was Director of Research and Chair of the Department of

Acupuncture at the New York College for Wholistic Health Education and Research (now the New York College for Health Professions).

Howard Hall holds two doctorate degrees in psychology, a PhD in experimental psychology from Princeton University and a PsyD in clinical psychology from Rutgers University. He is boarded in biofeedback and is an approved consultant in clinical hypnosis. Dr. Hall has conducted research and taught hypnosis at Pennsylvania State University and at Case Western Reserve University School of Medicine. He is currently an associate professor in the Department of Pediatrics, at the Case Medical Center and on staff at Rainbow Babies and Children Hospital in Cleveland, Ohio. For the past two decades Dr. Hall has conducted and published pioneering work on the effects of hypnosis, imagery, and relaxation on immune responses.

Donald McCown MSS, MAMS, is a lecturer in the School of Health Professions at Thomas Jefferson University in Philadelphia, Director of Mindfulness at Work Programs at Jefferson's Mindfulness Institute, and maintains a practice in mindfulness-based psychotherapy. A social worker trained at Bryn Mawr College, he also holds a Master of Applied Meditation Studies degree from the Won Institute of Graduate Studies, and has completed the most advanced teacher training in MBSR at University of Massachusetts Medical Center. He is co-author of *Teaching Mindfulness: A Practical Guide for Clinicians and Educators*.

Hari Sharma, MD, DABP, FCAP, FRCPC, DABHM is Professor Emeritus and former Director of the Division of Cancer Prevention and Natural Products Research, Department of Pathology, College of Medicine, The Ohio State University; Chairperson of the Integrated Medicine Committee of the American Association of Physicians of Indian Origin; and has been named a Fellow of the National Academy of Ayurveda by the Ministry of Health and Family Welfare, Government of India. Dr. Sharma's career represents a synthesis of the modern-day knowledge of Western medicine and the ancient knowledge of the natural, comprehensive Vedic system of health care.

Kenneth G. Zysk is associate professor and head of the department of Indology at Copenhagen University. He received his DPhil from the University of Oslo and PhD from the Australian National University. He has been an Indian Council for Cultural Relations Distinguished Visitor to India, a Senior Fulbright Fellow to India, American Institute for Indian Studies Fellow, and a Wellcome Fellow in the History of Medicine in London, and has served as Director of Dharam Hinduja Center's Indic Traditions of Healthcare project at Columbia University and taught at New York University.

References

Alexander, C.N., Langer, E.J., Newman, R.I., Chandler, H.M. and Davies, J.L. (1989) "Transcendental Meditation, mindfulness and longevity: An experimental study with the elderly." *Journal of Personality and Social Psychology 57*, 950–964.

Alexander, C.N., Robinson, P., Orme-Johnson, D.W., Schneider, R.H. and Walton, K.G. (1994a) "The effects of Transcendental Meditation compared to other methods of relaxation and meditation in reducing risk factors, morbidity and mortality." *Homeostasis 35*, 243–264.

Alexander, C.N., Robinson, P. and Rainforth, M. (1994b) "Treating alcohol, nicotine, and drug abuse through Transcendental Meditation: A review and statistical meta-analysis." *Alcoholism Treatment Quarterly 11*, 13–87.

Alexander, F.M. (1910) *Man's Supreme Inheritance: Conscious Guidance and Control in Relation to Human Evolution in Civilization*. London: Methuen.

American Cancer Society (2010) *Cancer Prevention and Early Detection Facts and Figures 2010*. Atlanta: American Cancer Society.

American Heart Association (2007) *Statistical Fact Sheet—Miscellaneous, 2007 Update*. Available at: www.americanheart.org/downloadable/heart/1173881560405CAUSOFDTH07doc.pdf, accessed August 8, 2008.

Anderson, J.W., Liu, C. and Kryscio, R.J. (2008) "Blood pressure response to Transcendental Meditation: a meta-analysis." *American Journal of Hypertension 21*, 310–316.

Andrews, L.B., Stocking, C., Krizek, T., Gottlieb, L., Krizek, C., Vargish, T. and Siegler, M. (1997) "An alternative strategy for studying adverse events in medical care." *Lancet 349*, 309–313.

Ansha, N. (1991) *Principles of Sufism*. Fremont, CA: Asian Humanities Press.

Armstrong, K. (1993) *Muhammad: A Biography of the Prophet*. San Francisco, CA: HarperCollins.

Badawi, K., Wallace, R.K., Orme-Johnson, D.W. and Rouzere, A.M. (1984) "Electrophysiologic characteristics of respiratory suspension periods occurring during the practice of the Transcendental Meditation program." *Psychosomatic Medicine 46*, 267–276.

Benor, D. (2001) *Spiritual Healing: Scientific Validation of a Healing Revolution*. Southfield, MI: Vision.

Bergson, H. (ed.) (1911) *Creative Evolution*. New York, NY: Henry Holt and Company.

Berwick, D.M. and Leape, L.L. (1999) "Reducing errors in medicine." *British Medical Journal* 319, 136–137.

Bhishagratna, K.K. (trans.) (1983) *An English Translation of the Sushruta Samhita Based on Original Sanskrit Text*, 3 volumes, 1907–1916. Reprint. Varanasi, India: Chowkhamba Sanskrit Series Office.

Bondy, S.C., Hernandez, T.M. and Mattia, C. (1994) "Antioxidant properties of two Ayurvedic herbal preparations." *Biochemical Archives 10*, 25–31.

Castillo-Richmond, A., Schneider, R.H., Alexander, C.N., *et al.* (2000) "Effects of stress reduction on carotid atherosclerosis in hypertensive African Americans." *Stroke 31*, 568–573.

Chalmers, R.A., Clements, G., Schenkluhn, H. and Weinless, M. (eds) (1989a) *Scientific Research on Maharishi's Transcendental Meditation and TM-Sidhi Program: Collected Papers, Volume 2.* Vlodrop, The Netherlands: MVU Press.

Chalmers, R.A., Clements, G., Schenkluhn, H. and Weinless, M. (eds) (1989b) *Scientific Research on Maharishi's Transcendental Meditation and TM-Sidhi Program: Collected Papers, Volume 3.* Vlodrop, The Netherlands: MVU Press.

Chalmers, R.A., Clements, G., Schenkluhn, H. and Weinless, M. (eds) (1989c) *Scientific Research on Maharishi's Transcendental Meditation and TM-Sidhi Program: Collected Papers*, Volume 4. Vlodrop, The Netherlands: MVU Press.

Chishti, G.M. (1991) *The Book of Sufi Healing.* Rochester, NY: Inner Traditions International.

Cooper, M.J. and Aygen, M.M. (1978) "Effect of Transcendental Meditation on serum cholesterol and blood pressure." *Harefuah Journal of Israel Medical Association 95*, 1, 1–2.

Cooper, M.J. and Aygen, M.M. (1979) "A relaxation technique in the management of hypercholesterolemia." *Journal of Human Stress 5*, 24–27.

Cross, A.J., Leitzmann, M.F., Gail, M.H., Hollenbeck, A.R., Schatzin, A. and Sinha, R. (2007) "A prospective study of red and processed meat intake in relation to cancer risk." *PLoS Med 4*, 12, e325. doi:10.1371/journal.pmed.0040325.

Cullen, W.J., Dulchavsky, S.A., Devasagayam, T.P.A. *et al.* (1997) "Effect of Maharishi AK-4 on H2O2-induced oxidative stress in isolated rat hearts." *Journal of Ethnopharmacology 56*, 215–222.

Dash, B. (1980) *Fundamentals of Ayurvedic Medicine.* Delhi: Bansal.

Dash, B. and Kashyap, L. (1980) *Basic Principles of Ayurveda Based on Ayurveda Saukhyam of Todarananda.* New Delhi: Concept.

Dewey, J. (1922) *Human Nature and Conduct.* New York: Henry Holt.

Dileepan, K.N., Patel, V., Sharma, H.M. and Stechschulte, D.J. (1990) "Priming of splenic lymphocytes after ingestion of an Ayurvedic herbal food supplement: Evidence for an immunomodulatory effect." *Biochemical Archives 6*, 267–274.

Dileepan, K.N., Varghese, S.T., Page, J.C. and Stechschulte, D.J. (1993) "Enhanced lymphoproliferative response, macrophage mediated tumor cell killing and nitric oxide production after ingestion of an Ayurvedic drug." Biochemical Archives 9, 365–374.

Dogra, J. and Bhargava, A. (2005) "Lipid peroxide in ischemic heart disease: effect of Maharishi Amrit Kalash herbal mixtures." *Indian Journal of Clinical Practice 16*, 4, 54–57.

Dogra, J., Grover, N., Kumar, P. and Aneja, N. (1994) "Indigenous free radical scavenger MAK4 and 5 in angina pectoris: Is it only a placebo?" *Journal of Association of Physicians India 42*, 6, 466–467.

Dossey, L. (1993) *Healing Words.* New York: HarperSanFrancisco.

Dossey, L. (1996) *Prayer is Good Medicine.* New York: HarperSanFrancisco.

Dossey, L. (2001) *Healing Beyond the Body: Medicine and the Infinite Reach of the Mind.* Boston, MA: Shambhala.

Dwivedi, C., Agrawal, P., Natarajan, K. and Sharma, H. (2005) "Antioxidant and protective effects of Amrit Nectar tablets on Adriamycin- and cisplatin-induced toxicities." *Journal of Alternative Complementary Medicine 11*, 1, 143–148.

Dwivedi, C., Sharma, H.M., Dobrowki, S. and Engineer, F. (1991) "Inhibitory effects of Maharishi Amrit Kalash (M-4) and Maharishi Amrit Kalash (M-5) on microsomal lipid peroxidation." *Pharmacology, Biochemistry and Behaviour 39*, 649–652.

Eddington, A. (1974) *The Nature of the Physical World*. Ann Arbor, MI: University of Michigan Press.

Engineer, F.N., Sharma, H.M. and Dwivedi, C. (1992) "Protective effects of M-4 and M-5 on Adriamycin-induced microsomal lipid peroxidation and mortality." *Biochemical Archives 8*, 267–272.

Eppley, K.R., Abrams, A. and Shear, J. (1989) "Differential effects of relaxation techniques on trait anxiety: A meta-analysis." *Journal of Clinical Psychology 45*, 957–974.

Ergil, K.V. (1983) *A Discussion of the Three Roots of Tibetan Medicine in the Context of the Treatment of Rheumatism*. Bachelor's thesis, private publication, Santa Cruz, CA.

Ergil, K.V. (1993) *A Discussion of the Three Roots of Tibetan Medicine in the Context of the Treatment of Rheumatism*. Bachelor's Thesis. Private Publication: Santa Cruz.

Ergil, K.V. (2006) "Tibetan Medicine." In M.S. Micozzi (ed) *Fundamentals of Complementary and Integrative Medicine* (3rd edition).

Fatoohi, L. (2002) *Jihad in the Qur'an*. Kuala Lumpur, Malaysia: AS Noordem.

Fatoohi, L. and Al-Dargazelli, S. (1999) *History Testifies to the Infallibility of the Qur'an*. Kuala Lumpur, Malaysia: AS Noordem.

Fraser, G.E. (1999) "Associations between diet and cancer, ischemic heart disease, and all-cause mortality in non-Hispanic white California Seventh-day Adventists." *American Journal of Clinical Nutrition 70*, 3 (suppl.), 532S–538S.

Gelderloos, P., Ahlstrom, H.H.B., Orme-Johnson, D.W. *et al.* (1990) "Influence of a Maharishi Ayur-Vedic herbal preparation on age-related visual discrimination." *International Journal of Psychosomatics 37*, 25–29.

Haines, D.D., Varga, B., Bak, I. *et al.* (2010) "Summative interaction between astaxanthin, Ginkgo biloba extract (EGb761) and vitamin C in suppression of respiratory inflammation: A comparison with ibuprofen." *Phytotherapy Research* [Epub ahead of print].

Hanna, A.N., Sharma, H.M., Kauffman, E.M. and Newman, H.A.I. (1994) "In vitro and in vivo inhibition of microsomal lipid peroxidation by MA-631." *Pharmacology, Biochemistry and Behaviour 48*, 505–510.

Herron, R.E. and Cavanaugh, K.L. (2005) "Can the Transcendental Meditation program reduce the medical expenditures of older people? A longitudinal cost-reduction study in Canada." *Journal of Social Behaviour and Personality 17*, 415–442.

Herron, R.E. and Fagan, J.B. (2002) "Lipophil-mediated reduction of toxicants in humans: An evaluation of an Ayurvedic detoxification procedure." *Alternative Therapies in Health and Medicine 8*, 5, 40–51.

Hilton, J. (1933) *Lost Horizon*. London: Macmillan.

Inaba, R., Mirbod, S.M. and Sugiura, H. (2005) "Effects of Maharishi Amrit Kalash 5 as an Ayurvedic herbal food supplement on immune functions in aged mice." *BMC Complementary and Alternative Medicine 5*, 8, doi:10.1186/1472-6882-5-8.

Inaba, R., Sugiura, H. and Iwata, H. (1995) "Immunomodulatory effects of Maharishi Amrit Kalash 4 and 5 in mice." *Japanese Journal of Hygiene 50*, 4, 901–905.

Inaba, R., Sugiura, H., Iwata, H. *et al.* (1996) "Immunomodulation by Maharishi Amrit Kalash 4 in mice." *Journal of Applied Nutrition 48*, 1–2, 10–21.

Inaba R, Sugiura H, Iwata, H. and Tanaka, T. (1997) "Dose-dependent activation of immune function in mice by ingestion of Maharishi Amrit Kalash 5." *Environmental Health and Preventative Medicine 2*, 1, 35–39.

Infante, J.R., Torres-Avisbal, M., Pinel, P. *et al.* (2001) "Catecholamine levels in practitioners of the Transcendental Meditation technique." *Physiology and Behaviour 72*, 1–2, 141–146.

Janssen, G.W. (1989) "The application of Maharishi Ayur-Ved in the treatment of ten chronic diseases: A pilot study." *Ned Tijdschr Geneeskd 5*, 35, 586–594.

Jawer, M.A. with Micozzi, M.S. (2009) *The Spiritual Anatomy of Emotion: How Feelings Link the Brain, the Body, and the Sixth Sense*. Rochester, VT: Park Street Press.

Jayadevappa, R., Johnson. J.C., Bloom, B.S. *et al.* (2007) "Effectiveness of Transcendental Meditation on functional capacity and quality of life of African Americans with congestive heart failure: A randomized control study." *Ethnicity and Disease 17*, 1, 72–77.

Jevning, R., Anand, R., Biedebach, M. and Fernando, G. (1996) "Effects on regional cerebral blood flow of transcendental meditation." *Physiology and Behaviour 59*, 3, 399–402.

Jolly, J. (1977) *Indian Medicine*, trans. G.C. Kashikar. New Delhi: Munshiram Manoharlal.

Key, T.J., Thorogood, M., Appleby, P.N. and Burr, M.L. (1996) "Dietary habits and mortality in 11,000 vegetarians and health-conscious people: Results of a 17-year follow-up." *British Medical Journal 313*, 7060, 775–779.

Khan, H.I. (1983) *The Music of Life*. New Lebanon, NY: Omega.

Kuhn, T.S. (1970) *The Structure of Scientific Revolutions*, 2nd edn. Chicago, IL: University of Chicago Press.

Kwok, T.K., Woo, J., Ho, S. and Sham, A. (2000) "Vegetarianism and ischemic heart disease in older Chinese women." *Journal of the American College of Nutrition 19*, 5, 622–627.

Lad, V. (1990) *Ayurveda. The Science of Self-Healing*. Wilmot, WI: Lotus Press.

Lazarou, J., Pomeranz, B.H, and Corey, P.N. (1998) "Incidence of adverse drug reactions in hospitalized patients." Journal of the American Medical Association 279, 1200–1205.

Lee, J.Y., Hanna, A.N., Lott, J.A. and Sharma, H.M. (1996) "The antioxidant and antiatherogenic effects of MAK-4 in WHHL rabbits." *Journal of Alternative and Complementary Medicine 2*, 4, 463–478.

Leskowitz, E. (2005) "From biology to spirit: The multidimensional model of wound healing." *Seminars in Integrative Medicine 3*, 1, 21.

Levine, J.P. (1976) "The Coherence Spectral Array (COSPAR) and its application to the study of spatial ordering in the EEG." *Proceedings of the San Diego Biomedical Symposium 15*, 237–247.

Meulenbeld, G.J. (1974) *The Madhavanidana and its Chief Commentary*. Leiden, Germany: Brill.

Micozzi, M.S. (1991) "Disease in antiquity: The case of cancer." *Archives of Pathology and Laboratory Medicine 115*, 838–844.

Micozzi, M.S. (1998) "Complementary medicine: What is appropriate? Who will provide it?" *Annals of Internal Medicine 129*, 65–66.

Micozzi, M.S. (2007) *Complementary and Integrative Medicine in Cancer Care and Prevention*. New York: Springer.

Misra, N.C., Sharma, H.M., Chaturvedi, A., Ramakant, S.M., Natu, J., Bogra, S.S. *et al.* (1994) "Antioxidant adjuvant therapy using a natural herbal mixture (MAK) during intensive chemotherapy: Reduction in toxicity—a prospective study of 62 patients." In R.S. Rao, M.G. Deo and L.D. Sanghvi (eds) *Proceedings of the XVI International Cancer Congress*. Bologna, Italy: Monduzzi Editore.

Mulacz, W.P. (1998) "Deliberately caused bodily damage (DCBD) phenomena: A different perspective." *Journal of the Society for Psychical Research 62*, 434–444.

Nader, T. (2000) *Human Physiology: Expression of Veda and the Vedic Literature*. Vlodrop, The Netherlands: MVU Press.

Nadkarni, A.K. (1908) *Dr. K. M. Nadkarni's Indian Materia Medica*, 3rd edn. Reprint. Bombay (Mumbai): Popular Prakashan.

Niwa, Y. (1991) "Effect of Maharishi-4 and Maharishi-5 on inflammatory mediators—with special reference to their free radical scavenging effect." *Indian Journal of Clinical Practice 1*, 23–27.

Orme-Johnson, D.W. and Farrow, J.T. (eds) (1977) *Scientific Research on the Transcendental Meditation program: Collected Papers*. Vol. 1. Rheinweiler, W. Germany: MERU Press.

Orme-Johnson, D.W. (1987) "Medical care utilization and the Transcendental Meditation program." *Psychosomatic Medicine 49*, 493–507.

Orme-Johnson, D.W. and Walton, K.G. (1998) "All approaches to preventing or reversing effects of stress are not the same." *American Journal of Health Promotion 12*, 5, 297–299.

Patel, V.K., Wang, J., Shen, R.N., Sharma, H.M. and Brahmi, Z. (1992) "Reduction of metastases of Lewis lung carcinoma by an Ayurvedic food supplement in mice." *Nutrition Research 12*, 667–676.

Patwardhan, B., Joshi, K. and Chopra, A. (2005) "Classification of human population based on HLA gene polymorphism and the concept of Prakriti in Ayurveda." Journal of Alternative Complementary Medicine 11, 349–353.

Penza, M., Montani, C., Jeremic, M. *et al.* (2007) "MAK-4 and -5 supplemented diet inhibits liver carcinogenesis in mice." *BMC Complementary and Alternative Medicine 7*, 19, doi:10.1186/1472-6882-7-19.

Planck, M. (1931) *The Observer,* 25 January.

Prasad, K.N., Edwards-Prasad, J., Kentroti, S. *et al.* (1992) "Ayurvedic (science of life) agents induce differentiation in murine neuroblastoma cells in culture." *Neuropharmacology 31*, 599–607.

Prasad, M.L., Parry, P. and Chan, C. (1993) "Ayurvedic agents produce differential effects on murine and human melanoma cells in vitro." *Nutrition and Cancer 20*, 79–86.

Rein, G. (2004) "Bioinformation within the biofield: Beyond bioelectromagnetics." *Journal of Alternative and Complementary Medicine 10*, 1, 59–68.

Rodella, L., Borsani, E., Rezzani, R. *et al.* (2004) "MAK-5 treatment enhances the nerve growth factor–mediated neurite outgrowth in PC12 cells." *Journal of Ethnopharmacology 93*, 161–166.

Rosano, L., Cianfrocca, R., Spinella, F. *et al.* (2010) "Combination therapy of zibotentan with cisplatinum and paclitaxel is an effective regimen for epithelial ovarian cancer." *Canadian Journal of Physiology and Pharmacology 88*, 6, 676–681.

Rubik, B. (2002) "The biofield hypothesis: Its biophysical basis and role in medicine." *Journal of Alternative and Complementary Medicine 8*, 6, 703–717.

Rumi, J. (1991) *Feeling the Shoulder of the Lion.* Putney, VT: Threshold Books.

Said, E. (1978) *Orientalism.* New York: Pantheon.

Salerno, J.W. and Smith, D.E. (1991) "The use of sesame oil and other vegetable oils in the inhibition of human colon cancer growth in vitro." *Anticancer Research 11*, 209–216.

Sannella, L. (1976) *The Kundalini Experience: Psychosis or Transcendence.* Lower Lake, CA: Integral Publishing.

Schneider, R.H., Nidich, S.I., Salerno, J.W. *et al.* (1998) "Lower lipid peroxide levels in practitioners of the Transcendental Meditation program." *Psychosomatic Medicine 60*, 38–41.

Sen Gupta, K.N. (1984 [1906]) *The Ayurvedic System of Medicine.* Reprint. New Delhi: Logos Press.

Sharma, P.V. (trans.) (1981–1994) *Caraka-Samhita. Agnivesha's Treatise Refined and Annotated by Caraka and Redacted by Dridhabala,* 4 volumes. Varanasi, India: Chaukhamba Orientalia.

Sharma, H.M. (1993) *Freedom from Disease: How to Control Free Radicals, a Major Cause of Aging and Disease.* Toronto: Veda Publishing.

Sharma, H.M. (2004) "Ayurvedic concept of Ama (toxin accumulation)." *AAPI Journal,* May/June, 29–30.

Sharma, H.M. (1997) "Phytochemical synergism: Beyond the active ingredient model." *Alternative Therapies in Clinical Practice 4*, 3, 91–96.

Sharma, H.M. (2002) "Free radicals and natural antioxidants in health and disease." *Journal of Applied Nutrition 52*, 2–3, 26–44.

Sharma, H.M., Dwivedi, C., Satter, B.C. and Abou-Issa, H. (1991) "Antineoplastic properties of Maharishi Amrit Kalash, an Ayurvedic food supplement, against 7,12-dimethylbenz(a) anthracene-induced mammary tumors in rats." *Journal of Research and Education in Indian Medicine 10*, 3, 1–8.

Sharma, H.M., Dwivedi, C., Satter, B.C. *et al.* (1990) "Antineoplastic properties of Maharishi-4 against DMBA-induced mammary tumors in rats." *Pharmacology, Biochemistry and Behaviour 35,* 767–773.

Sharma, H.M., Feng, Y. and Panganamala, R.V. (1989) "Maharishi Amrit Kalash (MAK) prevents human platelet aggregation." *Clinica and Terapia Cardiovascolare 8,* 227–230.

Sharma, H.M., Hanna, A.N., Kauffman, E.M. and Newman, H.A.I. (1992) "Inhibition of human LDL oxidation in vitro by Maharishi Ayur-Veda herbal mixtures." *Pharmacology, Biochemistry and Behaviour 43,* 1175–1182.

Sharma, H.M., Hanna, A.N., Kauffman, E.M. and Newman, H.A.I. (1995) "Effect of herbal mixture Student Rasayana on lipoxygenase activity and lipid peroxidation." *Free Radicical Biology and Medicine 18,* 687–697.

Sharma, H.M., Nidich, S.I., Sands, D. and Smith, D.E. (1993) "Improvement in cardiovascular risk factors through Panchakarma purification procedures." *Journal of Research and Education in Indian Medicine 12,* 4, 2–13.

Singh, R.H. (1992) *Pañchakarma Therapy.* Varanasi, India: Chowkhamba Sanskrit Series Office.

Sinha, R., Cross, A.J., Graubard, B.I. *et al.* (2009) "Meat intake and mortality." *Archives of Internal Medicine 169,* 6, 562–571.

Smith, C.W. (1998) "Is a living system a macroscopic quantum system?" *Frontier Perspect 7,* 9–15.

Smith, C.W. (2003) "Straws in the Wind." *Journal of Alternative and Complementary Medicine 9,* 1, 1–6.

Smith, C.W. (2011 in press) "Qi and the Frequencies of Bioelectricity." In D.M. Mayor and M.S. Micozzi (eds) *Energy Medicine East and West: A Natural History of Qi.* Edinburgh and London: Elsevier-Churchill Livingstone.

Smith, D.E. and Salerno, J.W. (1992) "Selective growth inhibition of a human malignant melanoma cell line by sesame oil in vitro." *Prostaglandins, Leukotrienes and Essential Fatty Acids 46,* 145–150.

Song, Y., Manson, J.E., Buring, J.E. and Liu, S. (2004) "A prospective study of red meat consumption and type 2 diabetes in middle-aged and elderly women." *Diabetes Care 27,* 2108–2115.

Srikanta Murthy, K.R. (trans.) (1984) *Sharngadharasamhita of Shrangadhara.* Varanasi, India: Chaukhamba Orientalia.

Srivastava, A., Samaiya, A., Taranikanti, V. *et al.* (2000) "Maharishi Amrit Kalash (MAK) reduces chemotherapy toxicity in breast cancer patients." *Federation of American Societies for Experimental Biology Journal 14,* 4, A720 (abstract).

Starfield, B. (2000) "Is US health really the best in the world?" *Journal of the American Medical Association 284,* 4, 483–485.

Sundaram, V., Hanna, A.N., Lubow, G.P. *et al.* (1997) "Inhibition of low-density lipoprotein oxidation by oral herbal mixtures Maharishi Amrit Kalash-4 and Maharishi Amrit Kalash-5 in hyperlipidemic patients." *American Journal of Medical Science 314,* 5, 303–310.

Svoboda, R.E. (1984) *Prakruti. Your Ayurvedic Constitution.* Albuquerque, NM: Geocom.

Thorogood, M., Mann, J., Appleby, P. and McPherson, K. (1994) "Risk of death from cancer and ischaemic heart disease in meat and non-meat eaters." *British Medical Journal 308,* 1667–1670.

Travis, F. and Arenander, A. (2006) "Cross-sectional and longitudinal study of effects of Transcendental Meditation practice on interhemispheric frontal asymmetry and frontal coherence." *International Journal of Neuroscience 116,* 1519–1538.

Travis, F., Haaga, D.A., Hagelin, J. *et al.* (2010) "A self-referential default brain state: Patterns of coherence, power, and eLORETA sources during eyes-closed rest and Transcendental Meditation practice." *Cognitive Processing 11,* 1, 21–30.

Upadhyay, S.D. (1986) *Nadivijana (Ancient Pulse Science).* Delhi: Chaukhamba Sanskrit Pratisthan.

Van Wijk, E.P.A., Koch, H., Bosman, S. and Van Wijk, R. (2006) "Anatomic characterization of human ultra-weak photon emission in practitioners of Transcendental Meditation and control subjects." *Journal of Alternative Complementary Medicine 12*, 1, 31–38.

Vang, A., Singh, P.N., Lee, J.W. *et al.* (2008) "Meats, processed meats, obesity, weight gain and occurrence of diabetes among adults: Findings from Adventist Health Studies." *Annals of Nutrition and Metabolism 52*, 2, 96–104.

Vohra, B.P., Sharma, S.P. and Kansal, V.K. (2001a) "Effect of Maharishi Amrit Kalash on age-dependent variations in mitochondrial antioxidant enzymes, lipid peroxidation and mitochondrial population in different regions of the central nervous system of guinea pigs." *Drug Metaolbolism and Drug Interactions 18*, 1, 57–68.

Vohra, B.P.S., James, T.J., Sharma, S.P. *et al.* (2002) "Dark neurons in the ageing cerebellum: Their mode of formation and effect of Maharishi Amrit Kalash." *Biogerontology 3*, 347–354.

Vohra, B.P.S., Sharma, S.P. and Kansal, V.K. (1999) "Maharishi Amrit Kalash rejuvenates ageing central nervous system's antioxidant defence system: An in vivo study." *Pharmacological Research 40*, 6, 497–502.

Vohra, B.P.S., Sharma, S.P. and Kansal, V.K. (2001b) "Maharishi Amrit Kalash, an Ayurvedic medicinal preparation, enhances cholinergic enzymes in aged guinea pig brain." *Indian Journal of Experimental Biology 39*, 1258–1262.

Vohra, B.P.S., Sharma, S.P., Kansal, V.K. and Gupta, S.K. (2001c) "Effect of Maharishi Amrit Kalash, an Ayurvedic herbal mixture, on lipid peroxidation and neuronal lipofuscin accumulation in ageing guinea pig brain." *Indian Journal of Experimental Biology 39*, 355–359.

Walborn, S.P. (2002) "Double-slit quantum erasure." *Physics Review A 65*, 1.

Walborn, S.P. (2003) "Quantum Erasure." *American Scientist 91*, 336.

Waldschütz, R. (1988) "Influence of Maharishi Ayur-Veda purification treatment on physiological and psychological health" [translation]. *Erfahrungsheilkunde Acta Medica Empirica 11*, 720–729.

Wallace, R.K. (1970) "Physiological effects of Transcendental Meditation." *Science 167*, 1751–1754.

Wallace, R.K., Dillbeck, M.C., Jacobe, E. and Harrington, B. (1982) "The effects of the Transcendental Meditation and TM-Sidhi program on the aging process." *International Journal of Neuroscience 16*, 53–58.

Wallace, R.K., Orme-Johnson, D.W. and Dillbeck, M.C. (eds) (1989) *Scientific Research on Maharishi's Transcendental Meditation and TM-Sidhi Program: Collected Papers*, Volume 5. Fairfield, IA: MIU Press.

Willett, W.C., Stampfer, M.J., Colditz, G.A., Rosner, B.A. and Speizer, F.E. (1990) "Relation of meat, fat and fiber intake to the risk of colon cancer in a prospective study among women." *New England Journal of Medicine 323*, 1664–1672.

Wittfogel, K.A. (1963) *Oriental Despotism: A Comparative Study of Total Power*. London and New Haven: Yale University Press.

World Health Organization (WHO) (2002) *WHO Traditional Medicine Strategy, 2002–2005*. Geneva: WHO.

Zysk, K.G. (1991) *Asceticism and Healing in Ancient India. Medicine in the Buddhist Monastery*. New York: Oxford University Press.

Zysk, K.G. (1993) *Religious Medicine: The History and Evolution of Indian Medicine*. New Brunswick, NJ: Transaction.

Zysk, K.G. (2000 [1991]) *Asceticism and Healing in Ancient India*. Delhi: Motilal Banarsidass.

Further Reading

Abdalati, H. (1996) *Islam in Focus*. Plainfield, IL: American Trust Publications.

Alter, J. (2004) *Yoga in Modern India: The Body Between Science and Philosophy*. Princeton, NJ: Princeton University Press.

Alter, J. (ed.) (2005) *Asian Medicine and Globalization: Encounters with Asia*. Pennsylvania, PA: University of Pennsylvania Press.

Arnold, T. and Guillaume, A. (1931) *The Legacy of Islam*. Oxford: Oxford University Press.

Avicenna (1993) *Al-Qanoon fi tibb (The Canon of Medicine)*. New Delhi: Dept. of Islamic Studies, Jamia Hamdard.

Bakar, O. (1990) "The philosophy of Islamic medicine and its relevance to the modern world." *MAAS Journal of Islamic science 6*, 1, 39–58.

Bernal, M. and Black, A. (1987) *The Afroasiatic Roots of Classical Civilization*. New Brunswick, NJ: Rutgers University Press.

Bucknell, R. S. and Stuart-Fox, M. (1993) *The Twilight Language: Explorations in Buddhist Meditation and Symbolism*. Richmond: Curzon Press.

Chishti, G.M. (1991) *The Traditional Healer's Handbook: A Classic Guide to the Medicine of Avicenna*. Rochester, VT: Healing Arts Press.

Deal, W.E. (2007) *Handbook to Life in Medieval and Early Modern Japan*. Oxford: Oxford University Press.

Dongden, Y. and Hopkins, J. (2003) *Health Through Balance: An Introduction to Tibetan Medicine*. Ithaca, NY: Snow Lion Publications.

Goldsmidt, A. (2008) *The Evolution of Chinese Medicine: Northern Song Dynasty 960-1200*. New York: Routledge.

Harper, D. (1998) *Early Chinese Medical Literature: The Mawangdui Medical Manuscripts*. London and New York: Kegan Paul.

King, H. (2001) *Greek and Roman Medicine*. London: Duckworth Publishers.

Korotkov, K. (2002) *Human Energy Field: Study with GDV Bioelectrography*. Fair Lawn, NJ: Backbone.

Korotkov, K. (2004) *Measuring Energy Fields: State-of-the-Science*. Fair Lawn, NJ: Backbone.

Kuriyama, S. (1999) *The Expressiveness of the Body and the Divergence of Greek and Chinese Medicine.* New York: Zone Books.

Levey, M. and Khaledy, N. (1967) *The Medical Formulary of Al-Samarqandi and the Relation of Early Arabic Simples to those Found in the Indigenous Medicine of the Near East and India.* Pennsylvania, PA: University of Pennsylvania Press.

Liebenskind, C. (1995) "Unani Medicine of the Subcontinent" in *Oriental Medicine: An Illustrated Guide to the Asian Arts of Healing.* Edited by Jan Van Alphen and Anthony Aris.

Lings, M. (1977) *What is Sufism?* Berkeley, CA: University of California Press.

Muhaiyaddeen, M.R.B. (1991) *Questions of life, answers of wisdom by the contemporary Sufi M.R. Bawa Muhaiyaddeen.* Volume 1. Philadelphia: Fellowship Press.

Munshi, Y., Ara, I., Rafique, H. and Ahmad, Z. (2008) "Leeching in the history—a review." *Pakistan Journal of Biological Science 11,* 13, 1650–1653.

Narayanaswami, V. (1975) *Introduction to the Siddha System of Medicine.* Madras: Pandit S.S. Anandam Research Institute of Siddha Medicine.

Natarajan, K. (2004) "'Divine Semen' and the Alchemical Conversion of Iramatevar." *The Medieval History Journal 7,* 2, 255–278.

Niranjana, D. (2006) *Medicine in South India.* Chennai: Eswar Press.

Nunn J. (2002) *Ancient Egyptian Medicine.* Oklahoma, OK: University of Oklahoma Press.

Osborn, D.K. (2008) *Greek Medicine.* Available from www.greekmedicine.com.

Oschman, J. (2000) *Energy medicine: the scientific basis.* London: Churchill Livingstone.

Porter, R. (1999) *The Greatest Benefit to Mankind: A Medical History of Humanity.* New York, NY: W.W. Norton & Company.

Rahimi, S.Y., McDonnell, D.E., Ahmadian, A. and Vender, J.R. (2007) "Medieval neurosurgery: contributions from the Middle East, Spain, and Persia." *Neurosurgery Focus 23,* 1, E14.

Rockwell, I. (2002) *The Five Wisdom Energies: A Buddhist Way of Understanding Personalities, Emotions, and Relationships.* Boston: Shambhala.

Scharfe, H. (1999) "The doctrine of the three humours in traditional Indian medicine and the alleged antiquity of Tamil Siddha medicine." *Journal of the American Oriental Society 119,* 4, 609-636.

Scheid, V. (2002) *Chinese Medicine in Contemporary China: Plurality and Synthesis.* Durham and London: Duke University Press.

Schipper, K. (1993) *The Taoist Body.* Berkeley, CA: University of California Press.

Shanmugavelan, A. and Sundararajan, A. (eds) (1992): *Siddhar's Source of Longevity and Kalpa Medicine in India.* Madras: Directorate of Indian Medicine and Homoeopathy.

Sivin, N. (1993) "Huang ti nei ching Suwen" in *Early Chinese Texts: A Bibliographical Guide.* Michael Loewe (ed.) Berkeley and Los Angeles: University of California Press.

Sivin, N. (1995) "State, Cosmos, and Body in the Last Three Centuries B.C." in *Harvard Journal of Asiatic Studies 55,* 1, 5–37.

Subramania, S.V. and Madhavan, V.R. (1984) *Heritage of the Tamils: Siddha Medicine.* Madras: International Institute of Tamil Studies.

Unschuld, P.U. (2003) *Huang Di Nei Jing Su Wen: Nature, Knowledge, and Imagery in an Ancient Chinese Medical Text.* Berkeley, CA: University of California Press.

Uthamaroyan, C.S. and Anaivaari R. Anandan (eds) (2005): *A Compendium of Siddha Medicine.* Chennai: Department of Indian Medicine and Homoeopathy, Government of Tamil Nadu.

Venkatraman, R. (1990) *A History of the Tamil Siddha Cult.* Mandurai: N.S. Ennes Publications.

Walford, R.L. (1983) *Maximum Life Span.* New York: Avon Books.

Woodward, M.R. (1985) "Healing and morality: a Javanese example." *Social Science and Medicine 21,* 1007–1021.

Yang, Shou-Zhong (ed/trans) (1998) *The Divine Farmer's Materia Medica: A Translation of the Shen Nong Ben Cao Jing.* Boulder, CO: Blue Poppy Press.

Zvelebil, K.V. (2003) *The Siddha Quest for Immortality.* Oxford: Mandrake of Oxford.

Subject Index

227

Author Index